Drug Addiction Research and the Health of Women

Executive Summary

Editors:
Cora Lee Wetherington, Ph.D., Women's Health Coordinator
Adele B. Roman, M.S.N., R.N., Deputy Women's Health Coordinator

U.S. DEPARTMENT OF HEALTH AND HUMAN SERVICES
National Institutes of Health

National Institute on Drug Abuse
5600 Fishers Lane
Rockville, MD 20857

Two publications have been produced based on the scientific research conference "Drug Addiction Research and the Health of Women," which was held on September 12-14, 1994, in Tysons Corner, VA, and was sponsored by the National Institute on Drug Abuse. This volume, *Drug Addiction Research and the Health of Women: Executive Summary*, contains condensed versions of the conference presentations as well as the ensuing discussion sessions. A companion volume, *Drug Addiction Research and the Health of Women*, builds on the conference presentations and provides greatly expanded reviews of research in this field.

To obtain copies of either publication contact the National Clearinghouse for Alcohol and Drug Information (NCADI), P.O. Box 2345, Rockville, MD 20847-2345, 1-800-NCADI-64 (622-3464) or see its World Wide Web site: http://www.health.org.

COPYRIGHT STATUS

DISCLAIMER

National Institute on Drug Abuse
NIH Publication No. 98-4289
Printed May 1998

Foreword

Alan I. Leshner, Ph.D.

Drug abuse and addiction are among the most pressing health and social issues facing our Nation, posing serious health risks and often tragic consequences for those who are afflicted and for their families and communities. Although extraordinary progress has been made in understanding these disorders and in finding the best ways to prevent and treat them, unfortunately, research on drug abuse and addiction related to women has, until relatively recently, been sorely neglected. Most drug abuse interventions developed to date, including prevention and treatment programs, have largely been shaped by men's characteristics and needs. Because women traditionally have been underrepresented in research studies and drug abuse treatment groups, the effects of drug abuse are far less understood for women than for men. But the scientific evidence generated thus far suggests that drug abuse and addiction present different challenges to women's health, progress differently in females than in males, and may require different treatment approaches and strategies. Moreover, the rapid increase in AIDS cases among women in recent years makes it all the more critical to address gender differences as they relate to drug problems.

In an effort to assess and begin to fill the gaps that exist in knowledge about drug abuse and women's health, the National Institute on Drug Abuse (NIDA), the Federal agency leading the Nation's research efforts on drug abuse and addiction, sponsored a national conference in September 1994 titled "Drug Addiction Research and the Health of Women." This 2-day meeting brought together leading researchers to present state-of-the-science findings, discuss research issues and challenges confronting the field, and lay the framework for NIDA's research agenda in this important area.

This volume contains condensed versions of the conference presentations as well as the ensuing discussion sessions. These summaries and discussions emphasize the gaps in knowledge regarding women and drug abuse that existed then and that, unfortunately, continue to exist today.

A companion volume, *Drug Addiction Research and the Health of Women*, contains greatly expanded reviews of research in this field.

Alan I. Leshner, Ph.D.
Director
National Institute on Drug Abuse
Parklawn Building, Room 10-05
5600 Fishers Lane
Rockville, MD 20857

For sale by the U.S. Government Printing Office
Superintendent of Documents, Mail Stop: SSOP, Washington, DC 20402-9328
ISBN 0-16-049570-9

Contents

Opening Session

WELCOME AND OPENING REMARKS

Loretta P. Finnegan, M.D.
Senior Adviser on Women's Issues
Office of the Director
National Institute on Drug Abuse

Dr. Finnegan explained the purposes of the conference: (1) discuss the status of research on drug addiction and women's health and learn about recent research findings and (2) determine what important research questions have not been answered and what questions should be given priority for future research. She encouraged participants to give NIDA written suggestions about what NIDA's research priorities should be and how its research agenda can be changed to improve the situation of women who suffer from drug addiction.

WELCOME FROM THE OFFICE OF RESEARCH ON WOMEN'S HEALTH

Vivian W. Pinn, M.D.
Associate Director for Research on Women's Health
Office of Research on Women's Health

Dr. Pinn greeted the conference participants on behalf of the Office of the Director at the National Institutes of Health (NIH) and the Office of Research on Women's Health (ORWH). Established in 1990, ORWH serves as the focal point for biomedical and behavioral research that addresses issues of sex differences across NIH. ORWH promotes a multidisciplinary approach to research that examines women's health across the lifespan.

ORWH's Basic Mandates

Dr. Pinn described ORWH's three basic mandates:

1. To determine what is known and not known about women's health. ORWH identifies priority issues and establishes the NIH research agenda on women's health, which includes stimulating

1

research on conditions that affect both women and men, but until now have been studied primarily in men, as well as diseases and conditions unique to women.

2. To fulfill the congressional mandate, codified in the NIH Revitalization Act of 1993, to ensure the inclusion of adequate numbers of women of diverse racial, ethnic, and socioeconomic backgrounds in NIH-supported clinical studies. To monitor inclusion across the entire NIH, a computer-based system has been established to track the inclusion of women and racial and ethnic minorities in clinical trials. Because inclusion raises important ethical and legal issues, ORWH commissioned a study by the Institute of Medicine (IOM) to define the implications of including women in clinical trials, especially women of childbearing age and potential. The resulting IOM report upheld the importance of inclusion, stating that, "women and men should have the opportunity to participate equally in the benefits and burdens of research."

3. To create and direct initiatives that will increase opportunities for women to pursue biomedical careers and to assume positions of leadership in biomedical research and participate in formulating public policy in this area.

ORWH's Research Agenda

- Published in 1992, ORWH's comprehensive research agenda *Opportunities for Research on Women's Health* is based on an expanded definition of women's health, one that addresses health across the lifespan and goes beyond reproductive issues. The agenda includes a broad range of scientific disciplines; medical specialties; and psychosocial, behavioral, and environmental factors. ORWH encourages future research to merge the study of biological and behavioral issues whenever possible.

- ORWH's agenda identified several research topics related to drug abuse, including (1) the link between drug abuse and neurobiological abnormalities; (2) the interaction among biological, psychological, and social factors that lead to harmful behaviors such as drug abuse; (3) the patterns and mechanisms of drug abuse, including drug addiction, by adolescent females; and (4) the influence of sex roles and relationships with male partners.

- One top research priority that ORWH has supported with supplemental funding is examination of behavioral and cultural factors related to women and disease risk or intervention. These factors include drug abuse, unsafe sexual behavior, domestic violence, and other abuse of elderly persons.

- The ORWH agenda stresses the need to include all populations of women in clinical research, including women from different racial and ethnic minority groups, socioeconomic statuses, sexual orientations, and geographic locations.

NIH is required by law to include women and members of racial and ethnic minority groups and subgroups in all federally funded clinical research using human subjects. In clinical trials with humans, it is necessary to include these groups so that valid data analyses can reveal any differences in interventions between the sexes and among racial and ethnic subgroups. ORWH constructed guidelines to help implement the law and has sought a balance between the requirement to include women as research subjects and the policies to protect them from potential risks.

WELCOME FROM THE NATIONAL INSTITUTE ON DRUG ABUSE

Alan I. Leshner, Ph.D.
Director
National Institute on Drug Abuse

Dr. Leshner presented a brief summary of NIDA's approach to research on drug abuse and women's health:

- NIDA views drug addiction as a chronic and relapsing disease that affects both women and men. Although most research on drug abuse has used men as research subjects, drug abuse may present different challenges to women's health, may progress differently in women than in men, and may require different treatment approaches.

- At the time of the conference, more than 4.4 million women had used an illicit drug at least once in the past month, and almost half of all women ages 15 to 44 years had used illicit drugs at least once in their lives. In 1991 NIDA established a Women's Health Issues Group to help focus research on women, initially on maternal-fetal interactions. Although the effects of drug abuse on pregnancy are still a priority, NIDA has broadened its research to examine the effects of drug abuse on all phases of women's lives.

- More attention is needed on the relationship between AIDS and drug abuse and how a patient's sex may affect this relationship. Drug abuse increases the risk of AIDS for women, especially women who inject drugs, share drug paraphernalia, or have sexual relationships with injection drug users. In the past few years, there has been a significant rise in the number of AIDS cases occurring in women who are injection drug users.

Dr. Leshner encouraged conference attendees to advise NIDA about research questions they believe should be prioritized and the most effective approaches for obtaining answers to those questions.

WELCOME FROM THE U.S. PUBLIC HEALTH SERVICE

Susan J. Blumenthal, M.D., M.P.A.
Deputy Assistant Secretary for Health (Women's Health)
Assistant Surgeon General
Office on Women's Health
U.S. Public Health Service

Women's Health and Drug Abuse

Drug abuse is a major contributor to premature morbidity and mortality in the United States. The annual direct and indirect costs of drug abuse total more than $58 billion. The Center on Addiction and Substance Abuse at Columbia University found that drug abuse and addiction are responsible for at least 20 percent of the $40 billion medicaid budget. Despite the widespread concern about addictive disorders in the United States, relatively little is known about the causes, treatment, and prevention of drug abuse disorders among women. Approximately 200,000 women are expected to die of illnesses related to drug abuse in 1994, more than four times the number of women who will die of breast cancer.

Society's denial about women and drug abuse is finally ending. Efforts to understand, treat, and prevent drug abuse are being strengthened at NIH since the 1992 ADAMHA Reorganization Act, which brought NIDA, the National Institute on Alcohol Abuse and Alcoholism, and the National Institute of Mental Health under the auspices of NIH. The reorganization has placed mental illness and addictive disorders, as critical elements of our national research agenda, side by side with cancer and heart disease. This is a major step forward in shattering the stigma that has surrounded addictive disorders.

Women's Health Research Issues

- Because of general improvements in public health, women's average life expectancy has increased by almost 30 years since 1900, and women live an average of 7 years longer than men. However, they now face—in greater numbers than men—the health problems that accompany old age, such as osteoporosis, depression, and Alzheimer's disease, and suffer from more illnesses and more chronic, debilitating conditions than men. Generations of physicians have not been trained about how diseases manifest differently in women or how to be sensitive to women's health concerns.

- Biomedical research has historically neglected research on women's issues, and most previous studies have been conducted with men only, with the results generalized to women. Research on drug addiction often has not been conducted with female subjects. Whereas women of childbearing age sometimes were excluded from medical research because of fear of damaging the fetus, the exclusion often reflected a social bias. In studies of everything from the link between smoking and cataracts to the benefits of aspirin for lowering the risks of a heart attack, the subjects have been all men.

- Women and men have different physiological responses to medications and drugs and may develop different manifestations of disease as a product of drug abuse. Women have more side effects and more fatal drug reactions to psychotropic medications

5

than men, but little research has been done in this area. Sex differences in weight, body composition, cerebral blood flow, gastric emptying time, and use of the exogenous hormones in oral contraceptives and estrogen replacement therapy may cause differences in drug reactions.

- Many individual genetic, biological, environmental, and psychosocial factors affect health and disease in men and women. Research has just begun to focus on sex-based differences in the morbidity of addictive disorders. Women suffer from illnesses and disabilities related to drug abuse that in the past were associated only with men, as well as disorders that appear to be unique to women.

- Most studies of drug abuse among women have centered on the effects of women's addiction on children and families, particularly on the fetus. These concerns reflect the traditional view that women are valued primarily for their reproductive capacity, but there has been a change in this philosophy and in the focus on women's health within the U.S. Department of Health and Human Services (DHHS).

Effects of Omitting Women From Research

- Major heart disease and cancer studies found smoking to be a major risk factor, but because they were conducted with only male participants, all smoking prevention trials have targeted men. However, in 1985 lung cancer surpassed breast cancer as a cause of death among women in the United States. Smoking also contributes significantly to other cancers in women—of the larynx, oral cavity, esophagus, and cervix—and contributes to impaired fertility, early menopause, pregnancy complications, and birth defects. Tobacco also interacts with other drugs such as oral contraceptives, markedly increasing the risk for cardiovascular disease among women.

- The complex psychosocial and biological reasons behind smoking behavior and cessation among women have not been evaluated and may complicate efforts to reduce the high rate of smoking among women. Approximately 25 percent of women younger than age 25 smoke cigarettes, and 23 percent of the adult female population are heavy smokers.

- The lack of research on how diseases manifest or can be prevented in women has led to increases in the rate of HIV infection. AIDS is the number one cause of death of reproductive-age women in many major cities. As many as 65.6 percent of the cases of HIV infection among women can be attributed to injection drug use or sex with an injection drug user.

- Young women use alcohol and other drugs at slightly higher rates than ever before and are at risk for drug abuse-related motor vehicle accidents and suicidal behavior.

- The incidence of polypharmacy (mixing medications for other than the intended purpose) is high among older women. Although elderly women represent only 11 percent of the population, they receive more than 25 percent of all written prescriptions—2-1/2 times more than those received by elderly men. Little research has been conducted on this high-risk population of women.

- Social sanctions and stigma against drug abuse among women have made them less willing to seek treatment for addictive disorders. As a result, data on the incidence and prevalence of drug abuse among women, generally based on contact with treatment facilities or help hotlines, may underrepresent the magnitude of the problem.

- Little awareness exists among health care professionals about sociocultural and environmental risk factors for women, particularly those affecting racial and ethnic minority groups. Environmental factors include sexual and other physical abuse, anxiety from having multiple roles as caregivers and wage earners, poor self-esteem, dead-end employment or unemployment, low educational attainment, and life stresses such as divorce and loneliness. How these factors may predispose women to drug abuse and what protective factors may exist remain unknown.

- In 1990 women's health began to receive unprecedented attention in both scientific circles and the media. The public and scientists have become aware of the exclusion of women from previous clinical trials, the inequity of access to health care services for women, the inadequate attention to health care and research-related sex differences, and the lack of women in senior medical positions in research and clinical practice.

Goals and Priorities of the Office on Women's Health

The U.S. Public Health Service's Office on Women's Health (PHS OWH) coordinates research, service delivery, and education programs across the agencies of DHHS, including NIH, the Food and Drug Administration, the Substance Abuse and Mental Health Services Administration, and others. PHS OWH is addressing crucial women's health issues and redressing inequities in the health care system that have compromised women's health. PHS OWH has the following goals:

- To support comprehensive, community-based health promotion and disease prevention programs for women, to improve access to health care services for women, and to promote healthier behaviors and lifestyles. Research shows that behavioral changes can reduce premature death by 70 percent and acute illnesses by more than 30 percent.

- To foster and sustain a comprehensive program of research on women's health issues.

- To support the training of health care professionals in women's health issues. PHS OWH is collaborating with NIH and the Health Resources and Services Administration to develop a model women's health curriculum for the training of health care professionals.

- To foster the promotion and advancement of women in health care and research careers.

THE HISTORY OF DRUG ABUSE AND WOMEN IN THE UNITED STATES

Stephen R. Kandall, M.D.

Abstract

Dr. Kandall presented a brief summary of the history of drug abuse and women in the United States. Although the news media may imply that drug abuse is a recent development, marijuana was brought by Jamestown settlers to the United States in the 17th century, and opiates were widely used during the Revolutionary War to control pain and diarrhea. Women made up the majority of drug users during the 19th century, and for the past 150 years, women, compared with men, have been overmedicated by physicians.

Although women have represented a large portion of the drug-using population in the United States, research on and treatment of drug abuse among women has received relatively little attention. Antidrug legislation has been promoted throughout U.S. history by linking drug abuse to prostitution and to public fears of racial and ethnic minority groups. In the past 25 years, there has been much progress in research and advocacy on women and drug abuse, but negative attitudes toward drug abusers have slowed this process. Women now represent approximately 30 percent of the drug-using population; this figure would be significantly higher if prescription drugs were included.

Introduction

Drug abuse as a health and social problem was first identified in 1850, but the extent and severity of drug abuse in society have never been determined. By 1900 the number of opiate addicts in the United States was estimated at 200,000, most of them women. Women usually took these drugs as laudanum (tincture of opium), paregoric (camphorated tincture of opium), and gum or powdered opium. Heroin was introduced in 1898 primarily as a cough suppressant, but because it was taken orally, which weakens its effect, heroin was not used widely in the late 19th and early 20th centuries.

Medicinal Use of Opiates and Cocaine in the 18th and 19th Centuries

The heavy use of opiates and the high rate of addiction in the 19th century were due largely to the way medications were used. Physicians and pharmacists had limited therapeutic options at their disposal, especially for treating pain and diarrhea. For example, during the Civil War, almost 3 million ounces of opium were distributed to the Union forces alone, and many wounded Civil War veterans became addicted. Almost all diseases were treated with opiates, including cholera, food poisoning, gallstones, headaches, rheumatism, pneumonia, asthma, consumption, cardiac conditions, syphilis, rabies, gangrene, earaches, hemorrhoids, and impotence.

The overmedication of women compared with men has been a major issue for the past 150 years, beginning with the image of the Victorian woman as less able to bear pain than a man and therefore more in need of medication. The typical drug addict during this period was a white, upper class woman from the South. Almost all anecdotal reports and epidemiologic studies written during the Victorian period cited gynecologic problems as the major reason for opiate treatment and addiction in women. Another major factor contributing to drug use in women during the late 19th century was neurasthenia, a condition of chronic physical and mental weakness that was said to be caused by exhaustion of the nervous system. Women were considered to be more susceptible to neurasthenia than men and were treated regularly with opiates.

Cocaine was introduced in the United States in 1876 and became a popular ingredient in many tonics and beverages, such as Coca-Cola, which contained the drug until it was replaced with caffeine in 1906. Cocaine also was used as a topical anesthetic for children and as a treatment for neurasthenia and was recommended as a treatment for opiate and alcohol addiction. Cannabis was prescribed widely between 1840 and 1900 for many conditions. In women it was prescribed for gynecologic problems, labor pains, postpartum psychoses, gonorrhea, and headaches.

The link between drugs and sexuality is another theme that has persisted over the past 150 years. Many images in the press showed women as helpless slaves to the opium habit and being lured into prostitution with drugs.

Drug Use at the Turn of the Century

By 1890 drug use had peaked and began to decrease by 1900, in part due to the changing sociodemographics of the United States. Physicians were becoming aware of the fact that drugs could be dangerous, and opiates were used less frequently to treat women's diseases.

In the late 19th and early 20th centuries, women from all economic classes formed the majority of opiate addicts in the United States and were prominent users of the "four Cs": chloroform, chloral hydrate, cocaine, and cannabis. At the same time, sectors of the U.S. pharmaceutical industry concentrated on developing and supplying drugs to women who were opiate addicts. Women were medicated disproportionately for physical, mental, and emotional complaints, but Victorian society would not acknowledge the existence of their drug problems.

Advances in public health and newer and safer analgesics made the use of opiates less acceptable, and physicians became aware of the risks of drug use during pregnancy. The 1865 standard gynecology textbook by William Byford recommended that amenorrhea be treated with opium, but the 1898 edition stated, "He who is compelled to resort frequently to opium must be considered devoid in diagnostic ability, and consequently ought not to be entrusted with the management of such cases." Mothers were held increasingly accountable for the inappropriate administration of opiates to their children, although in previous years opiates had been prescribed routinely for the treatment of many childhood illnesses.

Another major development at the turn of the century was the passage of antidrug legislation to control racial and ethnic minority groups who were seeking economic and social expansion, specifically Asian immigrants and blacks. Public fears of drug-induced attacks on women by racial and ethnic minority groups were used to promote antidrug legislation. In 1909 the international Shanghai Commission made it easier to move ahead with national antidrug legislation, claiming that "cocaine is often the direct incentive to the crime of rape by the Negroes of the South and other sections of the country," even though it had no evidence to support this claim. The perceived link between sexuality and drugs was strengthened by the increasing pervasiveness of the press and movies in everyday life.

The Harrison Act of 1914 was a watershed for antidrug legislation in the United States. It introduced repressive drug laws and reinforced negative attitudes toward drug abusers that persist today. The Harrison Act was a tax act that was not meant to restrict the use of narcotics but to tax their sale and track their flow. In 1919 the U.S. Supreme Court issued decisions that upheld the Harrison Act and prevented physicians from prescribing drugs solely for drug maintenance. The options available to drug addicts during this era were few. The first reported rise in crime among drug-addicted women occurred after passage of the Harrison Act. Between 1919 and 1923, the only organized treatments available were 44 drug treatment clinics scattered throughout the United States.

Drug Use and Drug Treatment Efforts in the 20th Century

Supporters of antimarijuana legislation promoted the image of women as potential victims of Mexican immigrants, which contributed to the passage of the Marijuana Tax Act of 1937. Just as opiates and cocaine were promoted in the 19th century, advertisements in the 1950s hailed the arrival of "happy pills," "peace-of-mind drugs," and "miracle drugs." In 1957 physicians wrote more than 48 million prescriptions for tranquilizers; by 1967 more than two-thirds of prescriptions for psychoactive drugs were written for women.

An attempt at organized drug abuse treatment by the Public Health Service can be found in the Lexington and Fort Worth "farms," which existed from the late 1930s to the early 1960s. In the late 1950s and early 1960s new drug treatment opportunities were offered in the form of outpatient and inpatient treatment, nonmaintenance treatment, and correctional treatment. Scientists pioneered methadone as another treatment option in the 1960s, and therapeutic communities were established.

The National Institute on Drug Abuse was founded in 1974. During the 1970s NIDA estimated that 1 million to 2 million women were addicted to prescription drugs, but physicians continued to write excessive numbers of prescriptions for women. In 1974, 22 million new prescriptions were written to provide Valium to women. Odyssey House, which opened in New York in 1966, was one of the first programs to offer care for pregnant addicts and their children with the support of a grant from NIDA.

Heroin use increased in the United States in 1970, and the proportion of female heroin addicts increased from about 18 to 30 percent. However, women were still underrepresented in drug treatment programs. The rate of arrests of women related to narcotics, larceny, theft, fraud, and forgery rose from 18 to more than 100 per 100,000 in only 10 years.

By 1971 President Nixon had declared drug abuse to be public enemy number one. The number of federally funded methadone programs grew from 16 in 1969 to 926 in 1973, with women making up almost 10,000 of the 42,000 methadone patients. However, these treatment programs did not address the multiple service needs of female addicts.

Public Law 94-371, passed in 1974, mandated special consideration for women in drug abuse prevention and treatment programs. During that same year, the Program for Women's Concerns was established within NIDA to address the lack of drug abuse treatment, prevention, and research programs for women. In 1975 NIDA began funding a series of 3-year comprehensive drug treatment demonstration projects for women in Detroit, Houston, New York, Philadelphia, Washington, DC, and San Raphael, CA, with an initial focus on treatment related to pregnancy.

In the 1980s and 1990s an impressive number of programs for drug-addicted women were created and implemented through the Public Health Service. For example, Congress designated a 5-percent set-aside for women's alcohol and other drug abuse treatment services for fiscal year 1986 (raised to 10 percent in 1989). These funds were channeled through an Alcohol, Drug Abuse, and Mental Health Services Administration (ADAMHA) block grant, which targeted services for pregnant women and women with dependent children. In 1988 ADAMHA funded the Pregnant and Postpartum Women and Infants demonstration grant program, which awarded 131 grants by the end of 1991. A variety of Government agencies began to operate programs for drug-addicted women, including the Office of the Assistant Secretary for Health, the Administration on Children and Families, the Administration for Native Americans, the Administration for Developmental Disabilities, and the Social Security Administration.

Even as women began receiving more treatment and prevention services, they also were blamed for certain health problems, including:

- An increase in the number of "crack babies" born, a term widely and indiscriminately used by the news media. Although there were widely differing estimates of the number of cocaine-exposed babies who were born during the 1980s and 1990s—from 100,000 to 375,000—the news media often reported the highest figures projected.
- A rise in perinatal AIDS because of transmission of HIV through the mother.
- Increased use of drugs by children.
- An increase in the incidence of congenital syphilis, a disease that was almost eradicated in the 1970s and early 1980s.

Punitive measures were taken against women who abused drugs. By April 1992 more than 160 women in 24 States had been prosecuted for drug use or drug-related behaviors during pregnancy. Racial bias was an important factor in determining who would be prosecuted. Dr. Ira Chasnoff, in his study of one Florida county, showed that even though drug use generally occurs equally across racial and ethnic groups, a member of a racial or ethnic minority group was 10 times more likely to be reported to child protective services than a white person.

Summary of Major Trends

- Throughout U.S. history, many drug abusers have been women. Before 1900 opiates and cocaine were standard treatments for many illnesses, including gynecologic problems. Women made up the majority of drug users during the 19th century and now make up about 30 percent of the total drug-using population. Historically, drug manufacturers have promoted images that portray women as weak and have marketed drugs to women to make a profit.

- Drug use and sexuality have been linked throughout U.S. history. Unfounded fears that drugs incite members of racial and ethnic minority groups to rape women have been used to promote antidrug legislation. The media have sensationalized stories about women's drug use, portraying women as victims of drug abuse or as mothers who allegedly abuse their children.

- Drug treatment for women received little attention until the 1970s. In the past 25 years, there has been much progress in research and advocacy on women and drug abuse. However, drug treatment is still relatively inaccessible for women. Persistent negative attitudes toward drug abusers have prevented progress in drug treatment.

Questions From the Audience

The question-and-answer session below followed Dr. Kandall's presentation.

Unidentified Audience Member: Have you encountered information specific to the epidemiology of drug abuse among women from racial and ethnic minority groups?

Dr. Kandall: Until the turn of the century, it was not discussed. Because much of the written epidemiology is contained in doctors' and pharmacists' records (I reviewed them as far back as the 1860s), minority groups are rarely mentioned. People who lived in rural or poor areas could not consult with physicians and tried to treat their own illnesses. However, as people and drugs moved to the inner cities, the problem of drug abuse among women in racial and ethnic minority groups became more serious. The analysis of the epidemiology of drug abuse has been poor, and even today, estimates vary about the number of drug addicts in different populations.

Unidentified Audience Member: It is important to know how many women and men are using drugs. For instance, we heard that 100,000 women were using opiates, but in addition to the absolute number, it is also important to know the proportions. For example, 100,000 out of 10 million women means something different from 100,000 out of 100 million. It also is important to know the age distribution. We need to understand the extent of the problem, the changes over time, and the distribution among different sectors of the population.

Dr. Kandall: Thank you very much.

Unidentified Audience Member: Would you like to speculate on what might have happened in the United States if there had not been groups of nonwhite people present who could be blamed for drug problems and be used to justify the passage of laws to limit drug use in this country? I am thinking of the United Kingdom, where people have been obtaining methadone on a regular basis since World War II. The number of nonwhite groups living in the United Kingdom is smaller than the number of racial and ethnic minority group members in the United States.

Dr. Kandall: That is a very provocative question. The major quantitative contribution to the drug problem was the medicinal use of drugs as prescribed by physicians and pharmacists and people who self-medicated because they had no access to physicians. There is no question that the numbers, which peaked in the 1890s, probably would have decreased anyway. I believe that the legislative agenda would have changed drastically if people from different racial and ethnic groups had not immigrated to the United States.

Unidentified Audience Member: In terms of the information that you have reported, it is interesting that the population groups that were targeted by antidrug legislation are the same groups that have serious drug problems and have no access to health care or drug treatment. As researchers, physicians, and health care providers, we need to look at creative ways of attacking and researching the problem; certainly, drug abuse prevention should be part of our approach.

Dr. Kandall: Thank you for that comment.

Unidentified Audience Member: I was struck by how similar the political motivations in the 1800s were to today's anti-abortion movement. I wonder if you came across any connections or parallels in your research.

Dr. Kandall: No, I have tried to write the book as a drug abuse history and not as a feminist tract. If there is information concerning that movement that you feel would be relevant, I would love to hear about it.

Unidentified Audience Member: I believe that one of the political bases for the anti-abortion movement was xenophobia because immigrants were reproducing more frequently than white women. Some people believed that outlawing abortion would increase the number of white infants who were born. There seems to have been a negative reaction to women using drugs in the same way that the anti-abortion movement reacted to the incipient women's movement.

Dr. Kandall: I guess the more things change, the more they stay the same.

Unidentified Audience Member: Would you give us some more background on how violence was tied to drug use, particularly the rape of women? I would like to know when that issue first emerged.

Dr. Kandall: It reached its apogee just prior to the Harrison Act when the so-called "cocaine-crazed blacks" allegedly were raping white women. Newspaper headlines on the subject were widely and boldly displayed. A side issue was the opium dens run by Chinese immigrants. It was not so much a matter of violence against women but the belief that women were being lured into prostitution with opium. The violence issue focused predominantly on blacks and was repeated to a lesser degree with the antimarijuana legislation brought on by the arrival of Mexican immigrants and their alleged sexual violence. Much of this was an attempt to control groups as they sought economic growth, and the issue of violence against women had no factual basis. An entire chapter in my book deals with the influence of movies and the major role played by these images of violence against women.

Unidentified Audience Member: Are you saying that there was an increase of violence against women or that this belief was a construction of the media?

Dr. Kandall: It was a construction of the media.

Unidentified Audience Member: What were some of the forces and events that triggered the news media's use of this theme and that helped to create an era of panic?

Dr. Kandall: The major issue, which you can read about in the testimony given before the U.S. House of Representatives, was the fear that women were becoming the victims of sexual predators from different racial and ethnic groups. The issue was raised to move antidrug legislation along more quickly, but there were no facts to back up this fear. One study of black cocaine users in Georgia who had been admitted to a particular hospital found that blacks had a much *lower* rate of sexual crimes than whites.

KEYNOTE ADDRESS: NEUROBIOLOGICAL CORRELATES OF THE ADDICTIONS: FINDINGS FROM BASIC AND TREATMENT RESEARCH

Mary Jeanne Kreek, M.D.

Abstract

Dr. Kreek presented information on the neurobiological basis of drug addiction and sex differences. Researchers have hypothesized that the endogenous opioid system may be involved in drug addiction and that multiple genes may contribute to the development of addictive and other diseases. Dr. Kreek proposed that more research is needed on the human opioid system, how it responds to different drugs, and sex differences. To improve efforts in drug abuse prevention, early intervention, and treatment, researchers must have a better understanding of the neurobiological basis of different drug addictions. Dr. Kreek stated that it is critical to combine laboratory studies and basic clinical research studies with applied treatment research to better understand the diseases of opiate, cocaine, and alcohol addiction.

Areas of Research

Dr. Kreek acknowledged the remarks of previous speakers regarding the critical importance of research on drug abuse and women, particularly because research has shown the correlation of drug abuse and HIV infection. She stated that the rapid rise of HIV infection among women makes it imperative to address the drug abuse problems of women at the prevention, early intervention, and treatment levels. In 1969 Dr. Kreek's laboratory began collecting blood samples from various studies of drug abusers in New York City. The researchers discovered that HIV began to appear in the blood of drug abusers in 1978.

In recent years, the New York City Department of Health has reported a high incidence of women infected with HIV, many through injection drug use or heterosexual contact with male injection drug users.

- One area of Dr. Kreek's research examines issues that help explain the neurobiological basis of drug addiction. Researchers suspect that multiple genes may contribute to the development of addictive diseases and other behavioral and physiological diseases. Vulnerability to drug addiction may exist when normal genes occur in specific combinations, but exposure to drugs is necessary also, thus making drug abuse prevention and early intervention particularly important.

- Data demonstrate that drugs of abuse alter normal human physiology, including stress response, reproductive biology, and immune function. Chronic diseases and responses to stressors may contribute to changing physiology, which also may increase vulnerability to drug addiction. These physiologic changes occur in both women and men and may contribute to other health problems. Many studies are in progress to determine whether the physiologic changes caused by drugs are persistent or permanent.

Role of the Endogenous Opioid System

- Dr. Kreek and others have been studying the role of the endogenous opioid system in heroin addiction, cocaine dependence, and alcoholism. The endogenous opioid system is involved in aspects of normal physiology-related stress response, reproductive biology, immune function, gastrointestinal function, cardiovascular status, and many behaviors, such as emotions and pain response. The three classes of endogenous opioid neuropeptides (peptides) are endorphins, enkephalins, and dynorphins.

- The partial structure of the opioid receptor gene is known, but not the complete five-prime sequences; many laboratories are studying the five-prime region in the gene because it controls how much of the gene message will be formed and therefore how much peptide will be produced. Two areas in the five-prime region are of special interest to scientists: (1) the area where stress-responsive steroids, like cortisone, bind to their receptors and act to change gene expression and (2) the area where estrogen and progesterone may act to change gene expression.

- One fundamental question being studied is whether there are differences between the sexes in gene expression because of the presence of differing amounts of estrogen and progesterone. Dr. Kreek's laboratory is conducting research with rodents to measure quantitatively how much gene message is expressed and to map where each opioid gene is expressed. There is gene expression in the hypothalamus, an area where there is neuroendocrine control both of stress response and reproductive biology.

- Scientists are trying to discover where and when gene expression for different opioid receptor genes (mu, delta, and kappa) occurs in the brain, how gene expression and receptor peptides are affected by drugs of abuse, and whether there are any sex differences. Mu and kappa opioid receptors are abundant in the regions of the brain where it is known that drugs of abuse act, as well as in the hypothalamus. New technology to image the human brain has made it possible to conduct studies in both those suffering from addictive diseases and those who are not addicted.

Pharmacotherapy for Opiate Addiction

- Early research on the treatment of heroin addiction led to a rationale and specific pharmacotherapeutic objectives for treating opiate addiction and other types of drug addiction: (1) prevent withdrawal symptoms such as those that occur with opiate dependence, (2) reduce drug craving, and (3) normalize any physiologic functions disrupted by drug abuse. To achieve these objectives, research should target the effect of treatment agents on specific sites of drug action, opiate receptors, or physiologic systems that have been affected or damaged by drug abuse.

- Methadone's pharmacokinetic profile is different from those of heroin and morphine and has a long-acting effect in humans. Dr. Kreek and her colleagues conducted a series of studies to analyze the action of methadone and determine whether there is any physical risk to addicts who use heroin while on methadone. They found that proper doses of methadone created tolerance to short-acting opiates like heroin and had no adverse or narcotic-like effects on the addict. Administering proper doses of metha-done creates greater tolerance for, and thus a blockage of, heroin's effects and allows normalization of disrupted physiology. Steady-dose methadone treatment does not create any narcotic effects, prevents withdrawal symptoms, and prevents the development of hunger for illicit opiates.

- Many studies have shown that highly significant reductions in the incidence of HIV infection occur among drug addicts who participate in effective methadone treatment programs.

- Dr. Kreek recommended that more access is needed to effective drug addiction treatment programs. In such programs, voluntary retention rates are from 70 to 85 percent, and continued use of heroin drops to less than 15 percent after stabilization (3 to 6 months in treatment). However, funding cuts in the past 20 years have reduced the ability of clinics to provide effective drug treatment and have reduced the availability of all types of treatment.

- Dr. Kreek asserted that an effective methadone program that combines drug abuse services with counseling and health care services would cost approximately $6,000 to $8,000 a year per individual. Although this is more than the current $1,500 to $3,500 a year often spent for pharmacotherapy, it is much less than the cost of treating end-stage AIDS (which has risen to $100,000 a year) or the cost of crime on the streets (up to $100,000 a year).

Neurobiological Correlates of Addictions

- The acute use of opiates and chronic use of short-acting opiates like heroin have been found to suppress the hormones of the hypothalamus, pituitary, adrenal (HPA) axis, which are involved in many physiological functions. Dr. Kreek found that during steady-dose methadone treatment, the HPA axis returned to normal and followed its normal rhythm of hormone release. Studies have found that patients on methadone experience a normalization of the reproductive biologic axis, the stress-responsive axis, and, in turn, the immune function that may be linked to the normalization of neuroendocrine function.

- Both cortisol and the endogenous opioid peptides are involved in the normal regulation of the HPA axis, and these opioids are regulated abnormally in individuals who are addicted to opiates and cocaine. New information reported by Dr. Kreek shows that opioid antagonists also activate the HPA axis, which has implications for the neurobiology of several addiction disorders, such as alcoholism. Activation of the HPA axis also may be important in explaining the small number of heroin addicts who have responded to treatment with naltrexone, an opiate antagonist.

- Basic clinical research has shown that the administration of acute doses of morphine or heroin affects humans differently than it does rodents. In humans, an injection of morphine causes the inhibition of the release of the adrenocorticotropic hormone, an important stress-responsive hormone, and beta endorphins. Opiates also inhibit the release of the luteinizing hormone that controls ovulation and testosterone levels.

- Acute doses of opiates also suppress or change the release of the glucocorticoid cortisol from the adrenal cortex. Recent research has examined where a glucocorticoid like cortisol, for example, dexamethasone, affects corticotropin-releasing factor (CRF). Dexamethasone affects CRF primarily in the hypothalamus, although researchers also have found CRF gene expression in other regions of the brain that may be involved in controlling emotions, behavior, and immune function.

- Acute use of opiates increases the release of prolactin, which modulates women's lactation and the immune system. Women in chronic methadone treatment have normal prolactin levels;

however, their prolactin levels increase modestly in response to peak plasma levels of methadone. The same was true in studies of women who were pregnant. During the second half of pregnancy, when prolactin levels normally increase dramatically, normally elevated prolactin levels were found in methadone-treated women. Because of the liver's enhanced ability to eliminate certain medications during pregnancy, plasma levels were significantly lower among methadone-treated women, even when the pregnant woman was maintained on a steady dose of methadone. After delivery, the woman's plasma level of methadone returned to what was considered normal. Physicians must be careful when considering any reduction in methadone dose during the late stages of pregnancy; methadone levels may be reduced even when the dose remains the same. Doses of methadone should not be lowered during the last two trimesters of a woman's pregnancy and should be maintained in a steady state to prevent the onset of drug withdrawal symptoms.

- Studies with rodents have shown that chronic cocaine administration increases the density of mu and kappa opioid receptors. Dr. Kreek's group has been trying to determine the role of dynorphin peptides in modulating the density of kappa opioid receptors, with the ultimate goal of discovering whether the natural endogenous opioid peptides can help decrease excess dopamine activity.

- Dynorphin peptides are potent modulators of prolactin release. Among healthy subjects, serum prolactin levels increased in direct response to dynorphin administration. In humans, prolactin is influenced almost exclusively by dopamine levels; therefore, Dr. Kreek and colleagues have suggested that dynorphin peptides may increase the release of prolactin by decreasing dopamine tone. This information may help researchers understand how to manage cocaine dependence.

- Heroin addicts are hyporesponsive to chemically induced stress, but former addicts maintained on methadone become normal in their response to such stress. Studies continue to investigate the relationship between stress and drug addiction. Drug-free, former heroin and cocaine addicts have been found to be hyperresponsive to chemically induced stress. Researchers now want to find out whether such hyperresponsiveness in drug-free, former heroin and cocaine addicts may drive them to readminister or begin using opiates.

- Studies of humans and rodents have shown that both endogenous and exogenous opiates (e.g., heroin) may alter specific indices of immune function. Dr. Kreek's group studied heroin addicts and former addicts who were maintained on moderate-to-high-dose methadone treatment for at least 11 consecutive years. Both groups had used injection drugs for a similar number of years, so it was assumed that both groups had been exposed equally to drug-related diseases. The heroin addicts, who were HIV-1 negative, were found to have abnormally high levels of CD4+ and CD8+ cells and lowered natural killer cell activity, which are all important for balancing the immune function and are disrupted by AIDS. However, the absolute number of cells was normal in the former addicts who had been in long-term treatment with methadone and had normal natural killer cell activity. Research on how drugs of abuse affect CD4+ and CD8+ cells is particularly important because these cells are the first line of defense against many diseases.

Issues for Future Research

- More research is needed on how different opioid receptors are affected by drugs of abuse and what sex differences may exist.
- In humans, prolactin is influenced almost exclusively by dopamine levels; therefore, Dr. Kreek and colleagues have suggested that dynorphin peptides may increase the release of prolactin by decreasing dopamine tone. More research in this area may help researchers understand how to manage cocaine dependence.
- Research should target the effects of specific treatments on specific sites of action, receptors, or physiologic systems that have been affected or damaged by the drug of abuse.
- Former heroin and cocaine addicts who are drug-free have been found to be hyperresponsive to chemically induced stress. Research is needed to determine whether such hyperresponsiveness may drive former addicts to readminister opiates.
- Research is needed on how drugs of abuse affect the activity of CD4+ and CD8+ cells and natural killer cells, which is

particularly important because these cells are the first line of defense against many diseases and may be related to the progression of AIDS.

Epidemiology

EPIDEMIOLOGY OF DRUG USE AND ABUSE AMONG WOMEN

Denise B. Kandel, Ph.D.

Abstract

Dr. Kandel's presentation dealt with the epidemiology of drug abuse involving two different paths of research: (1) examining patterns of drug abuse by individuals, including frequency of drug abuse, and (2) attempting to measure the extent of drug abuse by investigating behaviors and symptoms that meet the criteria for diagnosis of a drug abuse disorder. Dr. Kandel asserted that epidemiologic studies based on samples of the general population rather than on specific high-risk groups can better assess the distribution of drug abuse and the need for drug treatment services because such samples are free from selection and referral biases. She presented data on the epidemiology of drug use and drug abuse disorders from two national studies and data on the developmental patterns and consequences of women's drug use from the longitudinal cohort that she has followed from their adolescence to mid-thirties. There is a well-developed sequence from licit drug use to illicit drug abuse. Dr. Kandel's study revealed the intergenerational transmission of smoking and showed that cigarette smoking may play an important role in women's progression to illicit drug abuse. Dr. Kandel suggested that research involving a collaboration of disciplines, ranging from biology to psychology, may increase understanding of drug abuse behaviors.

Results of the 1992 National Household Survey on Drug Abuse

The National Household Survey on Drug Abuse collects information on drug use by individuals age 12 and older. Dr. Kandel presented data from the 1992 survey, the most recent one for which sex-specific data were available [at the time of this presentation], to illustrate three important points:

24

1. The prevalence of drug abuse differed markedly for different drugs, with prevalence highest for licit drugs. Among illicit drugs, marijuana was used most frequently, followed by cocaine. Illicit drugs include psychotherapeutic drugs used for nonmedical purposes.

2. Most abuse of both licit and illicit drugs occurred among young people between ages 12 and 34 and peaked during ages 18 to 25. As individuals grew older, their drug abuse declined, but more gradually with licit drugs than illicit drugs.

3. About 22 percent more males than females used drugs. Differences between the sexes in drug abuse seemed to increase with age. The level of drug involvement also differed between the sexes. For example, among high school seniors who had used cigarettes or other drugs daily, more than twice as many males as females also used alcohol and marijuana daily.

Results of the National Comorbidity Survey

Dr. Kandel also presented data from the National Comorbidity Survey, conducted by Professor Ronald Kessler of the University of Michigan, which provided the most recent data on the distribution of drug abuse disorders among the U.S. population. This survey was carried out in a representative sample of individuals ages 15 to 54. Professor Kessler's unpublished data indicated the following:

- There was more drug dependence and abuse of illicit drugs and alcohol by men than by women. Six percent of women ages 15 to 54 met the criteria for lifetime drug dependence. Of women who had ever used illicit drugs, 13 percent met the criteria for dependence, and of those who had used heroin, 25 percent met the criteria for heroin dependence.

- Women were dependent on cigarettes more than any other class of drugs. Tobacco (nicotine) may be the most addictive of any of the drugs studied. Thirty-one percent of women who had ever smoked met the criteria for dependence. There was a slight difference between women and men in the number who were dependent on tobacco smoking.

- More women than men were at risk of becoming dependent on psychotherapeutic drugs used nonmedically.

- There was much comorbidity among psychiatric disorders, and most comorbidity was alcohol-related. The most frequent class of psychiatric disorder diagnosed among women was anxiety; among men, the most frequent psychiatric disorder was related to conduct or use of drugs. Professor Kessler and his group were able to determine whether a drug abuse disorder was primary or secondary (whether it appeared before any other psychiatric disorders). In four out of five cases, a drug-related disorder was secondary to another psychiatric disorder.

Dr. Kandel argued that if drug abuse disorders occur secondarily to other psychiatric disorders, then prevention efforts should be emphasized when an individual first seeks treatment for the primary disorder. Drug abuse prevention and treatment efforts must be tailored with an understanding of the different disorders that are prevalent in women and men.

Studies of Developmental Stages of Drug Involvement

On the basis of studies by Dr. Kandel in the early 1970s on a cohort of individuals she followed for nearly 20 years, a well-developed sequence or progression from licit to illicit drug abuse was determined. Some of Dr. Kandel's findings were as follows:

- The first drug used was either alcohol or nicotine. Cigarettes seemed particularly important in females' progression to illicit drug abuse. For males, alcohol alone was sufficient to lead to use of illicit drugs, and cigarettes were not significant.
- The use of licit drugs in the early stage of drug abuse seemed necessary, but it was not the only factor for movement to the next stage of drug abuse. Therefore, the use of licit drugs at an early age, especially cigarettes, is important for predicting subsequent drug abuse and behaviors.
- If young people followed the sequence to using illicit drugs, the first illicit drug most tried was marijuana. Few people used other illicit drugs without experimenting first with marijuana.

Consequences of Drug Use by Women

These studies also revealed the health consequences of women's drug use:

- The age-specific rates of childbearing were compared with the age-specific rates of illicit drug use or heavy smoking (one pack a day). The age-specific rate of childbearing peaked at the point where there also was a high rate of illicit drug use.

- Interviews of mothers, fathers, and preadolescent children revealed intergenerational transmission of smoking behavior. Analysis of the tobacco-smoking behaviors of 192 mother-child pairs revealed that smoking during pregnancy was related to smoking by preadolescents, with a much stronger effect on girls than on boys. Multivariate analyses of the data controlled for current smoking, sociodemographic characteristics, and other variables, and results indicated that if the mother smoked during pregnancy, it was likely the daughter also would become a smoker. Dr. Kandel replicated this finding in a national sample of 804 mother-child pairs. Her data raise the possibility that nicotine or other tobacco components released by maternal smoking during a critical period of prenatal brain development might alter the brain response to the effects of nicotine later in life. Such changes may predispose a child, especially a female, to smoke and persist in smoking. Therefore, prenatal exposure to drugs may affect drug abuse behaviors that are not manifested for more than 10 years.

Issues for Future Research

- Collaboration among disciplines ranging from biology to psychology and sociology is needed for better understanding of drug abuse behavior. Women's dependence on nicotine may be the most important area to study, particularly because smoking may be transmitted from one generation to the next.

- As they grow older, more women than men meet the criteria for a diagnosis of drug dependence. Cultural and metabolic factors require further investigation.

Questions From the Audience

The question-and-answer session below followed Dr. Kandel's presentation.

Unidentified Audience Member: What is the possible relationship between depression in the mother and smoking by daughters? Could depression be a mediating variable?

Dr. Kandel: This is an important point that I plan to explore in future studies. We know there is a strong relationship between depression and smoking. There could be various physiological explanations, but it may be that women who persist in smoking are more depressed and have a genetic liability either to depression or to smoking. This may explain why transmission is stronger among females than among males.

Unidentified Audience Member: An alternative explanation could be the role-modeling of the smoking mother for the adolescent daughter. How did you rule that out as an alternate explanation?

Dr. Kandel: As I mentioned earlier, we included maternal current smoking in the multivariate logistic regressions, as well as other covariates, when we estimated the effect of prenatal smoking on off-spring smoking. In descriptive tabular analyses, we examined the children's smoking among four groups of women who had different combinations of current and prenatal smoking patterns. The results showed that the mother's current smoking had absolutely no effect on the daughter's smoking behavior, and that the prenatal effect was the most significant factor.

Unidentified Audience Member: What is the effect of the mother's smoking during the child's developmental stages rather than before birth? Were the intermediate stages of child development checked?

Dr. Kandel: We did not have enough cases to examine that differentiation, but we had continuous retrospective histories of smoking, so we created a measure that was a proportion of the child's life during which the mother was smoking. Although we could not do the refined analysis you suggest, this crude categorization of current smoking versus smoking during pregnancy captured the persistent smoking behavior and the child's length of exposure to the mother's smoking.

Biological/Behavioral Mechanisms

DRUG ABUSE AND REPRODUCTION IN WOMEN

Nancy K. Mello, Ph.D.

Abstract

Dr. Mello addressed the question of how alcohol, cocaine, opiates, and other drugs of abuse disrupt the functioning and regularity of the endocrine system and how such disruption may subsequently relate to menstrual cycle disorders and compromise other aspects of women's health. She and her colleagues studied the menstrual cycles of female rhesus monkeys, whose neuroendocrine control system is similar to that of human females; preliminary data suggest that cocaine and alcohol may stimulate release of an essential reproductive hormone, luteinizing hormone (LH), and also increase adrenocorticotropic hormone (ACTH), resulting in the disruption of the normal menstrual cycle and amenorrhea. These data complicate earlier assumptions about how cocaine may disrupt the menstrual cycle. More research is needed on how cocaine interacts with female reproductive hormones and prospects for recovery.

Menstrual and Reproductive Disorders

Alcohol, cocaine, opiates, and other commonly abused drugs have been associated with disruption of the menstrual cycle and compromising of female reproduction. Several major reproductive disorders may be associated with the interaction of hormones and drugs such as cocaine:

- Amenorrhea: complete cessation of menstruation for months or years
- Luteal phase dysfunction: a short luteal phase, consisting of 8 days or less from ovulation to menstruation; an inadequate luteal phase during which progesterone levels are abnormally low
- Anovulation: failure to ovulate
- Disorders of prolactin regulation: abnormally high levels of prolactin (hyperprolactinemia)
- Galactorrhea: a condition involving the abnormal secretion of breast milk, sometimes associated with hyperprolactinemia

- Spontaneous abortion: abortion that occurs naturally
- Ovulation is preceded by a surge in LH, and there is evidence that the LH pulsatile release gradually increases in amplitude and culminates in ovulation. Infrequent or absent LH pulses have been associated with fertility disorders and amenorrhea. The rhythm of the menstrual cycle is controlled in part by the rhythms of the pulsatile release of LH and follicle-stimulating hormone (FSH). In an anovulatory cycle, menstruation may occur, but there is no midcycle peak in LH and FSH.
- Preliminary data on monkeys suggest that cocaine and alcohol may disrupt pulsatile release of LH, resulting in disruption of the normal menstrual cycle and amenorrhea. It is not clear whether amenorrhea associated with chronic cocaine exposure is a consequence of cocaine's effects on LH; estradiol, which regulates LH release; or the regulation of prolactin.

Effects of Cocaine on the Menstrual Cycle

- Studies of rhesus monkeys reveal that administration of synthetic corticotropin-releasing factor (CRF) suppresses the release of LH and FSH, which can result in anovulation and amenorrhea. Emerging research data indicate that acute cocaine or alcohol intoxication may stimulate ACTH and stimulate rather than suppress the release of LH from the pituitary gland. These data complicate earlier assumptions about how cocaine may disrupt the menstrual cycle.
- Recent research has revealed that cocaine stimulates LH production in both female and male humans and rhesus monkeys; the only exception was ovariectomized female monkeys, in which cocaine had no effect. This information is unexpected because studies of pharmacologic actions have shown that administration of dopamine agonists suppresses rather than increases LH. Yet a significant increase in LH after acute cocaine administration has been a consistent, robust finding across species. The implications of a cocaine-induced increase in LH are unknown, but if cocaine increases LH levels near the middle of the menstrual cycle, this could trigger ovulation and result in an increased risk of pregnancy.

30

Hyperprolactinemia

- High levels of prolactin have often been associated with chronic cocaine abuse and withdrawal; however, the clinical implications are not clear.

- An acute dose of cocaine results in prolactin suppression, presumably by increasing dopamine levels. It is possible that chronic cocaine exposure impairs the regulatory relationship between the production of hypothalamic dopamine and prolactin. Some data suggest that a dopamine probe can reveal cocaine-related changes in prolactin regulation before the development of overt hyperprolactinemia.

- Hyperprolactinemia may contribute to menstrual cycle abnormalities and amenorrhea, compromise the immune system, and increase vulnerability to AIDS.

Sex Differences

- The presence of estradiol may be an important factor in whether cocaine stimulates LH or ACTH production. Researchers found that cocaine stimulated the production of LH and ACTH in both female and male humans and rhesus monkeys, with the exception of ovariectomized female monkeys who had only trace amounts of estradiol. Presumably, differences between the sexes in the biologic effects of drugs would reflect hormonal differences between women and men.

- There is a possibility that estrogens and progestins may protect women from cocaine-associated cerebral vasospasms. Estrogens may protect women from mild atherosclerosis, and after menopause, estrogen replacement therapy also has a protective effect and reduces women's risk for premature cardiac disease and osteoporosis. Research has revealed that cerebral perfusion abnormalities are common in cocaine abusers. One surprising discovery was found in a group of nine women and nine men who were cocaine abusers and were matched in terms of age. The women had fewer cerebral perfusion defects than the men, even though the women reported using cocaine for significantly longer periods than the men, an average of 15.0 years and 8.2 years, respectively. The investigators concluded that differences between the sexes in cerebral perfusion abnormalities could not be explained by differences in age, race, body mass index, level of alcohol or cocaine use, or route of drug administration.

Issues for Future Research

- It is not clear whether amenorrhea associated with chronic cocaine exposure is a consequence of cocaine's effects on LH; estradiol, which regulates LH release; ACTH, which may suppress LH release; or the regulation of prolactin. Studies are under way to examine the role of estradiol in cocaine's effects on LH, but more research is needed on cocaine's effects on reproductive hormones. What are the implications of cocaine-induced increases in LH and the possible effects on ovulation and the increased likelihood of pregnancy?

- Research is needed on the mechanisms that underlie cocaine's effects on prolactin regulation and the clinical significance of hyperprolactinemia.

- Future research should clarify how cocaine interacts with reproductive hormones to cause menstrual and other reproductive disorders. What is the effect of reproductive hormones influenced by cocaine on the functioning of the brain and the immune system?

Questions From the Audience

The question-and-answer session below followed Dr. Mello's presentation.

Dr. James Woods: Were you able to account for any weight changes that might have influenced the hormonal and menstrual abnormalities? Or did you not find any differences in weight during your research?

Dr. Mello: We did not find differences in weight. Your question is important because a number of things can be associated with amenorrhea. Inherent in your question is the fact that cocaine is known to have anorectic effects. The monkeys were allowed to self-administer food, so we had an objective measure of how much they took. We also supplemented that diet each day with fruit, vegetables, and monkey chow, and we recorded the weight about every 2 weeks. The monkeys developed tolerance to cocaine's anorectic effects rapidly, within about 2 weeks. The weight of the monkeys remained remarkably stable.

Unidentified Audience Member: Has anyone observed a relationship between the pattern of cocaine abuse by women and the use of hormonal contraceptives?

Dr. Mello: I do not know of any data or any study that directly addresses that question.

Unidentified Audience Member: In your research, have you noted any differences in the sexual arousal of females related to cocaine use? Is there any evidence of sexual arousal correlated with an increase in LH in women? Is cocaine-related sexual arousal most often reported by men or women?

Dr. Mello: We do not have direct observations of the sexual behavior or receptivity of female monkeys because they are housed individually. There is speculation that cocaine's stimulation of LH may be related to the sexual arousal that cocaine abusers report. Both men and women have reported sexual arousal related to cocaine use.

SEX DIFFERENCES, DRUGS, AND DEFENSIVE BEHAVIOR

D. Caroline Blanchard, Ph.D.

Abstract

Dr. Blanchard's presentation addressed sex differences in anxiety, depression, and defensive behaviors among humans and other animals and their relationship to drug abuse. She defined "defensive behavior" as a large number of actions taken by humans or other animals when they are threatened or traumatized by a painful or harmful event—actions such as flight, avoidance, freezing, defensive threat and attack, risk assessment, sonic vocalizations, and, in some species, ultrasonic mobilizations. She asserted that anxiety, depression, and defensive behaviors involve neurotransmitter and neuromodulator systems that operate differently in females and males. Almost no preclinical research has been conducted with female subjects on the effects of serotoninergic compounds. Dr. Blanchard asserted that these sex differences are too great to be ignored and should be studied because they are important factors in drug abuse.

Sex Differences Related to Anxiety, Depression, and Defensive Behaviors

- Anxiety and panic disorders are more prevalent among women than among men; agoraphobia is about three times as common among women. Some large community studies suggest that women account for as many as 70 to 75 percent of those suffering from posttraumatic stress disorder. Because women are diagnosed with anxiety and depression disorders more often than men, they are prescribed drugs more often to treat these disorders.

- Anxiety, depression, and other psychiatric conditions can promote abuse of mood-altering drugs, including alcohol and prescription and nonprescription medications. The use of alcohol in particular is viewed as an attempt to self-medicate. In one study of approximately 5,000 young adults, 22 percent abused alcohol and nonprescription drugs. Those who abused drugs suffered more from anxiety and depression than the average member of the group. In approximately 75 percent of the drug abusers, the onset of anxiety or depression preceded drug abuse, sometimes by a substantial period.

- Studies of the defensive behaviors of rats and mice have revealed some parallels with human behavior. Under conditions of great social stress, those animals that behave most defensively are the ones that demonstrate the greatest increase in alcohol consumption. Clinical studies in human subjects indicate that a family history of violence predicts alcohol abuse and spouse abuse by children when they grow older.

- Females of every mammalian species studied have exhibited more defensive behaviors than the males of the same species. A recent article revealed that the administration of testosterone to some female mammals dramatically reduced their defensive behaviors, suggesting that there is some biological basis for sex differences in these behaviors. Sex differences have been found in virtually all measures of defensive behaviors. The behaviors most responsive to anxiolytic drugs were also the ones that most differentiated male and female rats.

- Among both humans and laboratory animals, there are major sex differences in the neurotransmitter and neuromodulator systems.

34

The neurotransmitters are known to be involved in reactions to stress or threats of danger.

- Almost no preclinical research on the effects of serotoninergic compounds has been conducted with female subjects, or even with a mix of females and males. It is important to conduct preclinical research in psychopharmacology using female animals, given that the mechanisms of the serotonin system differ by sex. Serotoninergic medications are used to treat anxiety, and selective serotonin reuptake inhibitors are used to treat panic and depression. Because of the lack of knowledge about sex differences in the mechanisms and treatment of anxiety and depression, current treatment for those disorders is inadequate for both women and men. Dr. Blanchard speculated that researchers may have abandoned studies of treatments that did not show potential for male subjects but may have had potential for females.

- If anxiety and depression can be treated more effectively in women, then progress can be made in solving drug abuse problems that originate from the need to self-medicate or from exposure to medications for those disorders.

Issues for Future Research

- Evidence suggests that anxiety, depression, and defensive behaviors involve neurotransmitter and neuromodulator systems that operate differently in women and men. Because those systems are important factors in drug abuse, sex differences must be studied thoroughly.

- Dr. Blanchard speculated that more effective treatments for anxiety and depression might reduce the prevalence of drug abuse.

- Given that there are sex-related differences in the serotonin system and serotonin is linked to defensive behaviors, it is important to conduct preclinical research in psychopharmacology using nonhuman female animals. Almost no preclinical research has been conducted on the effects of serotoninergic compounds with female subjects. A special initiative is therefore needed to ensure that such research is conducted. Preclinical psychopharmacologic studies are the precursors to clinical trials, and therefore the research is necessary to discover the most effective treatments of anxiety and depression for women.

Questions From the Audience

The question-and-answer session below followed Dr. Blanchard's presentation.

Dr. Risa Goldstein: I am concerned that a lot of the research that has been discussed relies on retrospective recall to date the presence of mood disorders and defensive behaviors related to substance abuse. Given the inherent difficulties with retrospective recall, do you feel that caveats should be added to the information presented today?

Dr. Blanchard: Yes, there is good reason to insert a number of caveats. I examined the data from human research, but in most cases I am not qualified to analyze the data because my expertise is in animal research. However, as Dr. Kandel pointed out in her presentation, many people who abuse drugs also suffer from anxiety or some other psychiatric disorder; the degree of comorbidity is too high to be ignored. We should be cautious about drawing conclusions, but I believe that we gain insights from animal research. I encourage the integration of animal and human research and the recognition that the results of animal research are not irrelevant to human research. In many cases, the animal data can help to develop a firmer scientific foundation for the results of human research.

Dr. Zili Sloboda: I concur with what has been said about the problems inherent in research based on retrospective recall. We are learning that drug abuse is complex, and it is difficult to separate the individual factors involved. The presentations of Dr. Blanchard and others suggest the importance of developing studies that link human epidemiologic research with animal research.

Dr. Karla Moras: I want to highlight the points made by the last few speakers about the methodological difficulties in analyzing anxiety and mood disorders among chronic drug abusers. At the University of Pennsylvania, we are conducting a NIDA-funded multisite study of cocaine addiction. We find it extraordinarily difficult to determine what is a freestanding mood or anxiety disorder separate from the results of drug abuse.

Dr. Blanchard: I do not think anyone will disagree with that. The animal research provides hypotheses for the human work, as well as vice versa. For example, the concept of risk assessment in animals—highly motivated information-gathering—has led us to examine to what extent this is a feature of anxious individuals. We discovered that it is a definite feature of at least the clinical descriptions of many anxious individuals. We will not understand the value of this research until a lot more evidence is in.

Biological/Behavioral Mechanisms Panel

SEX DIFFERENCES AND HORMONAL EFFECTS ON DRUG SEEKING

David C.S. Roberts, Ph.D.

Abstract

Dr. Roberts presented background information on how the brain responds to cocaine and estrogen. Animal self-administration experiments are used to simulate the human condition and achieve better understanding of brain mechanisms. Such experiments can examine how the brain responds to drug reinforcement mechanisms and how brain systems are altered. The results of an experiment several years ago revealed that the estrous cycle of female rats affects their motivation to self-administer cocaine. Dr. Roberts discussed the implications for research on whether the human menstrual cycle can affect the drug-dependent behavior of women addicted to cocaine.

Background

- In Dr. Roberts' research, rats were given the opportunity to perform an action—usually to press a lever—that resulted in their receiving an intravenous injection of cocaine. The action of pressing the lever was used to measure the animal's drug-dependent behavior. Brain manipulations were performed to determine whether it was possible to affect the reinforcing actions of cocaine. The data revealed that there are a number of critical areas in the brain that could totally disrupt the rat's cocaine self-administration behavior.

- Researchers in Ann Arbor and Quebec have been studying the effects of the estrous cycle, estrogen administration, and ovariectomies on the behavioral responses of female rats. Their research has determined that female rats are more responsive than male rats to psychomotor and stimulant drugs. Treatment with estrogen usually increases the female rat's response to the drugs, and ovariectomies dampen the response.

- The rat's estrous cycle and treatment with estrogen affect the release of the brain's dopamine cells in response to amphetamines and other stimulants.

Findings on Cocaine Use and the Estrous Cycle

- If the animal was allowed to obtain a drug injection for each lever press, the animal consistently waited a specific period of time before repeating the lever press and obtaining the next injection; this behavior was dose-dependent.

- The motivation of the rats to obtain cocaine injections was measured by use of a progressive ratio schedule in which the number of times a rat had to press the lever before obtaining another injection increased exponentially. Male rats receiving low doses of cocaine would press the lever 300 times before giving up. As the dose of cocaine increased, the rats increased the number of times they were willing to press the lever before giving up.

- Female rats exhibited a similar drug-response behavior, but their motivation to respond was higher than that of males; they completed much higher ratios than males to obtain the same doses of cocaine. The drug-response behavior of female rats also was less consistent than that of male rats.

- To determine whether female rats self-administer cocaine differently during their 4- or 5-day estrous cycle, their behavioral inconsistency was analyzed. The analysis revealed that female rats exhibited different drug use behavior on just 1 day—the day of estrus—when they would go to enormous lengths to obtain an injection of cocaine, pressing the lever more than 600 times.

Future Research

Research is needed to determine whether the menstrual cycle has an important influence on women who are drug-dependent. Although it is known that the estrous cycle increases the motivation of female rats to self-administer cocaine, it is not known whether women's menstrual cycle can have a similar effect. Human experiments are needed to determine whether the menstrual cycle has a similar, motivating effect on women's drug-dependent behavior.

SMOKING, EATING, STRESS, AND DRUG USE: SEX DIFFERENCES

Neil E. Grunberg, Ph.D.

Abstract

Dr. Grunberg's presentation emphasized that sex differences are key issues in drug abuse research, particularly with regard to the interaction of drug use, smoking, eating, and stress. The interaction of these variables must be understood for researchers to address the biological mechanisms of drug abuse. Two-way interactions have been well researched, including studies of stress and eating, stress and drug use, sex differences and eating, and sex differences and drug use. There is a critical need, however, for research on three-way interactions that involve examining sex differences in drug use and simultaneously measuring the effects of two additional variables such as stress and smoking, stress and eating, or smoking and eating.

Stress

Stress and the use of illicit drugs, and licit drugs such as alcohol and tobacco, have been correlated in humans during drug initiation, maintenance, and relapse phases. The effects of psychological, perceptual, and cognitive strategies on drug use are important to reducing stress and treating drug abuse. Few studies have examined whether women and men can be influenced differently by the expectancy of drug effects and the cognitive variables that affect drug actions.

Smoking

The use of tobacco and nicotine has a significant effect on women's health, and it is critical that scientists understand how tobacco affects women and men differently. Twenty-five percent of women in the United States smoke. More young women smoke than young men, and the number of young women who smoke is increasing.

- Females, both humans and laboratory animals, are more sensitive to the actions of nicotine than are males, and females are more likely to respond to the toxic effects of high levels of nicotine.

- According to Dr. Grunberg's research, females are more sensitive to nicotine's effect on eating and body weight. Female rats have been shown to eat more and gain more weight when they quit using nicotine, and women are concerned about weight gain when they quit smoking.

Eating

- Dr. Grunberg suggested that drug abuse research include eating disorders. Many of the same mechanisms that regulate eating behaviors and eating disorders are common to drug addiction. He asserted that one's sex and one's eating behaviors interact and have powerful effects on drug use. Eating behaviors and responses can reveal the basic mechanisms of drug abuse and related sex differences. With more research, it may be possible to understand how different drugs cause drug dependence and eating disorders among females and males.

- Stress and eating disorders are related, and both have a powerful effect on drug use. Generally, men eat more than women, but stress affects eating behaviors among men and women in opposite ways. In mild, anxiety-provoking situations, women eat greater amounts of foods that are sweet and high in carbohydrates. In contrast, stress causes men to eat less food overall.

- Eating disorders, such as anorexia nervosa, bulimia, and overeating, are more common among women than among men.

Opiates and Alcohol

- Stress and opiate use also are correlated in humans, in terms of drug initiation, maintenance, and relapse; increases in stress increase the likelihood of opiate use. But the use of opiates in the general population is less frequent than the use of nicotine or alcohol. The discovery of sex differences in opiate effects dates back at least 10 years, but little work has been done to examine the effects of these relationships.

Dr. Grunberg's group conducted a series of studies that compared the drug administration response and stressors of female and male laboratory animals. The research revealed the following:

- As with nicotine, the interaction of opiates and stress had significantly different effects on females and males. Stress caused both female and male animals to self-administer more opiates, but females consumed more opiates than did males.

- There were sex differences in both alcohol use and its effect on the stress response. Women and men may drink while under stress but for different psychological or biological reasons.

Issues for Future Research

- Decisions and clarifications are needed on which drugs will be included or excluded in the national drug abuse research and public policy agenda. Will the research agenda focus exclusively on illicit drugs? Or will it also include tobacco and alcohol?

- Examination of stress is a critical element in drug abuse research. Stress can be used as an independent variable in studying different responses and revealing the underlying mechanisms of drug action.

- It is important to study how a person's sex interacts with different drugs and behaviors because the interactions usually reveal the most important and serendipitous information about the mechanisms at work.

- Hypotheses about the biological and behavioral interactions of drug use, stress, and sex can be developed and analyzed through use of nonhuman animal models and comparison of the results with information based on research with humans.

41

- Stress and cocaine use correlate, particularly with regard to drug relapse; more research is needed to examine sex differences in the interaction of cocaine and stress.

- It is critical to do additional research on three-way interactions, such as the interactions of sex differences and stress with use of alcohol, cocaine, opiates, nicotine, and other drugs. Such studies must examine sex differences at the same time they measure the effects of drug use, stress, smoking, or eating.

- More research is needed to examine the suggestion that the expectancy of drug effects and the cognitive variables that affect drug action may interact with stress and have different influences on women and men.

TRANSLATING BASIC RESEARCH INTO THE CLINICAL SETTING

James R. Woods, Jr., M.D.

Abstract

Dr. Woods emphasized that all obstetricians should be concerned about drug abuse because it is the most widespread problem in maternal-fetal medicine and high-risk obstetrics. Research is needed on drug-related questions that obstetricians have faced for years. His presentation focused on the progress of basic research on drug abuse and pregnancy, particularly the need for more research on cocaine use. There is preliminary evidence linking cocaine use with the unexpected deaths of pregnant women, and there are serious concerns about how cocaine affects a pregnant woman's uterine blood flow and the blood pressure and heart rate of the fetus. Many miscarriages and cases of premature labor have been linked to cocaine use. Dr. Woods noted that drug abuse is not unique to poor and medically underserved individuals; it involves individuals from all racial and ethnic groups. He acknowledged the difficulty of separating the problem of drug abuse from the poverty and violence that often accompany it and offered suggestions for improving the medical system's approach to caring for women addicted to drugs.

Effects of Cocaine Abuse on Pregnant Women

Dr. Woods described some observations that he and other researchers have made in the past few years about cocaine and its effect on the physiology of pregnant women.

- Cocaine stimulates a pregnant woman's heart and raises her blood pressure and heart rate, which subjects the fetus and delicate blood vessels in the placenta to unusual increases in blood pressure. The increases in maternal heart rate and blood pressure also create the need for an increase in blood flow and oxygen to the heart. However, cocaine has been shown, in nonhuman animals that were not pregnant, to restrict the increase in coronary blood flow that normally occurs when the heart rate and blood pressure rise. Although cocaine causes the heart rate and blood pressure to increase, it causes the blood flow in the uterus to decrease. There are serious concerns about what effects cocaine may have on the coronary blood flow of pregnant women. There is preliminary evidence linking cocaine use with unexpected deaths of pregnant women.

- Many miscarriages and cases of premature labor have been related to the use of cocaine during pregnancy. According to research in Michigan, chronic cocaine exposure may make the uterus unable to respond to beta-receptor agonists, the primary medication used to stop premature labor.

- Cocaine use by a pregnant woman raises the fetal blood pressure and heart rate. Several researchers have observed that cocaine crosses the placenta quickly, and within 2 minutes the cocaine levels in the fetus can equal those in the mother.

- Dr. Woods and his colleagues recently published reports on a study in which cocaine was instilled directly into the amniotic fluid of nonhuman animals that had not been exposed previously to the drug. Cocaine can enter the fetal circulatory system at about 3 to 5 percent of the cocaine concentrations in the amniotic fluid. The researchers believe that cocaine in the amniotic fluid can enter the fetal circulatory system through the placenta or the umbilical cord. They do not know whether amniotic fluid might act as a reservoir that could expose the fetus to cocaine long after a pregnant woman has stopped using the drug.

Approaches to Improving the Care of Women

Dr. Woods emphasized that efforts to reduce drug abuse and related health risks among women also must respond to other problems caused by poverty, violence, and socioeconomic issues. He asserted that drug abuse and approaches to treating it should be redefined; an improvement in medical care will fail to change the current situation unless there are increased efforts to connect women to the social services and medical care they need. He suggested several activities that clinics could implement to improve the care of women addicted to drugs:

- Increase outreach programs that complement the resources of the medical community. Such programs facilitate prenatal care and help build trust with women in the community. Some pregnant women who are addicted to drugs need assistance with solving basic problems such as obtaining social services or coping with the lack of transportation or a telephone.

- Link obstetrics with community residential drug treatment programs, mental health programs, intensive day treatment care, and outpatient care to help women who use drugs gain access to contraceptives and prenatal care.

- Address the distrust and fear felt by many pregnant women who are addicted to drugs. Many women avoid contact with the medical community because they are afraid their children will be taken away from them.

- Provide patients with continuity of care, an important factor in building trust; patients want to be able to see the same clinician each time they visit the clinic.

- Be more responsive to the practical problems and needs of the patients; make clinic procedures flexible enough to respond to patients who may have difficulty adhering to clinic rules and schedules. For example, rescheduling an appointment for a patient who arrives late rather than "fitting her in" may be very discouraging if the patient has little access to transportation.

Issues for Future Research

- Cocaine causes an increase in maternal heart rate and blood pressure, but it restricts the increase in coronary blood flow that should occur. More research is needed on how such restriction in blood flow affects pregnant women.

- Some evidence suggests that pregnancy may predispose a woman to enhanced cocaine cardiotoxicity. Additional research is needed to understand how cardiotoxicity affects pregnant women who use drugs.

- More research is needed on the relationship of cocaine use to miscarriage and premature labor. Alternative medications to prevent premature labor should be developed. Chronic cocaine use may reduce the effectiveness of beta-receptor agonists, the primary medications used to stop premature labor.

- Cocaine raises the fetal blood pressure and heart rate. Non-human animal research suggests that cocaine concentrations can be transferred from the mother to the fetus through the placenta or umbilical cord. More research is needed on the effects of maternal cocaine use on the fetus.

- Research is needed on drug-related questions that obstetricians have faced for years. For example, should women who are addicted to heroin go through drug detoxification during pregnancy? If so, how should the fetus be monitored during the process?

BIOLOGICAL/BEHAVIORAL
MECHANISMS PANEL DISCUSSION

The discussion presented below followed presentations by members of the Biological/Behavioral Mechanisms Panel: Drs. Roberts, Grunberg, and Woods.

Dr. Shirley Coletti: How can researchers use the information that NIDA has collected to better educate those who make decisions about the funding of drug treatment, including members of Congress, other legislators, and other decisionmakers? There is a tremendous focus now on the criminalization of drug abuse and funding the building of prisons rather than drug treatment. How can NIDA's information be used to educate people?

Dr. Woods: The only way to convince members of Congress of the need for funding of drug treatment is to remind them that drug abuse is truly a medical disease. Treatment of drug abuse is complex; it cannot be treated in the way that a simple pain can be treated with aspirin. In the next few years, the biggest challenge will be to prove that drug abuse treatment programs are effective and cost-efficient.

Dr. Loretta Finnegan: Research on mental health and drug abuse (of both licit and illicit drugs) has been integrated into NIH. Under the auspices of NIH, drug abuse clearly is defined as a health issue. However, educating people about drug abuse is a continuing struggle, and it is important to get information to the news media. Congress also needs education on the effect of advertising on drug abuse, particularly with regard to women.

Dr. Stephen Kandall: Part of the answer has to do with Dr. Grunberg's suggestion to reframe the dialog and redefine drug abuse. When drug abuse is viewed as a problem affecting a small number of people, money for treatment and research is not available. When AIDS was redefined as a disease affecting the large, white, heterosexual population, more money was made available for research. If drug abuse can be defined more broadly to include abuse of alcohol and nicotine, it is more likely to gain funding because it is an issue that is relevant to larger numbers of people.

Unidentified Audience Member: I want to comment on an area that has tremendous growth potential. The hospital-based studies of the American Society of Addiction Medicine have revealed that drug abuse is a major factor contributing to other health problems that patients first present at the hospital. We have tried to collaborate with colleagues in pediatrics, obstetrics, and psychiatry, and I think we need to do more of this. We also need more information about the cost of health care services related to drug abuse and its effect on the delivery of health care services in this country, particularly with regard to women.

Dr. Woods: It is an irony that cigarette smoking and alcohol use are clearly the greatest health problems in obstetrics, but screening for these substances usually is not done.

Dr. Kandall: But that has nothing to do with science; it reflects the political agenda that directs our work. Alcohol is far worse than any other drug I can think of in terms of the effects on the fetus and the newborn infant, but alcohol abuse is viewed differently from other drug abuse solely because of how society chooses to define drug abuse. If drug abuse continues to be viewed as a problem affecting just a small number of people rather than our whole society, then the definition of drug abuse will not be broadened and there will not be an increase in support for research and treatment.

Dr. Grunberg: One way to change the perspective of physicians about drug abuse is to influence the medical education of physicians. The best time to educate physicians is during their first year of medical school. If we explain to medical students at the beginning of their medical education that drug abuse, including abuse of nicotine and alcohol, is the single most preventable cause of death and illness, then they are more likely to maintain a broader view of drug abuse in their medical practices. Perhaps NIDA and others could persuade the accrediting boards, the American Medical Association (AMA), and particularly the American Association of Medical Colleges (AAMC) to require educating physicians about the effects of nicotine, alcohol, and other drug abuse. Many medical schools do not include drug abuse in their curriculums. I recently presented a paper at an international conference in Germany where we discussed how to improve the education of physicians around the world about the effects of tobacco.

Unidentified Audience Member: I want to comment on Dr. Woods' characterization of drug abuse as a chronic, relapsing disease. We may have enough evidence to conclude that drug abuse is a relapsing disorder, but I am concerned about using the word "disease" to define it. The concept of disease is a double-edged sword. On the one hand, it can relieve people of stigma, but on the other hand, it involves certain assumptions about etiology and potential treatment. The data presented here today do not lead to the conclusion that drug abuse is a disease, but they do indicate that there are environmental influences, such as psychosocial stressors, that affect people's use of drugs.

Dr. Finnegan: But one could say that also about heart disease. With the science that has been presented today, one can say clearly that drug abuse causes a disruption in the normal functioning of the brain and hormones. I think that we are getting closer and closer to defining drug abuse as a chronic, relapsing disease.

Dr. Woods: The point is well taken. For the most part, I use the term "disease" when referring to drug abuse because I want to convince my physician colleagues that they need to change their attitudes and approaches to drug abuse.

Dr. Risa Goldstein: Dr. Woods' recommendations concerning a kind of "one-stop shopping" and the availability of multiple services for pregnant and postpartum women really struck a chord with me. I did a study several years ago of contraceptive behavior among drug abusers during a 3-month period before they entered a drug detoxification program. The most striking finding was that 40 percent of both women and men who were heterosexually active (including those not known to be pregnant, postmenopausal, or surgically sterile) used no contraceptive method at all during that 3-month period. One facet of the medical management of chronic, relapsing conditions is the patient's responsibility for self-care and for planning life events, including pregnancies. How can we encourage female drug abusers to take more responsibility in this area?

Dr. Woods: We brought together a focus group of women and asked them that very question. It became instantly clear to us that these women are capable of determining when they are ready for a certain stage of drug treatment. Dr. Ira Chasnoff told me several years ago that you cannot place women into residential treatment unless they feel ready to work on their drug problem. Women do not enter residential treatment when they feel good about their lives; they choose to enter residential treatment when they are unhappy and have hit "rock bottom."

The issue of contraception should be raised immediately after women give birth. First, they have to be helped to adjust to the postpartum period so that they have more confidence about taking control of their health care and their sexuality. Then they can be helped to make decisions about contraceptive planning. I think Norplant and Depo-Provera are going to have an effect, particularly Depo-Provera. One side effect of Norplant is weight gain, and this is causing many women to discontinue use after about 6 months.

Dr. Finnegan: I want to address Dr. Grunberg's challenge to NIDA to research licit as well as illicit drugs. NIDA deals primarily with illicit drugs, but its research is not necessarily restricted to those drugs. Several years ago, NIDA developed a protocol that focused on maternal lifestyles and infant outcomes, and this study encompassed many of the issues that have been discussed today.

Mr. Richard Millstein: Different Government agencies are responsible for various aspects of research on drug abuse. Abuse of alcohol always has been separated from other forms of drug abuse. In many

States, alcohol abuse and other drug abuse are the responsibility of a single agency, but the Federal Government has a long history of keeping them separate. In the past few years, NIDA has looked at expanding its research on nicotine addiction, and we have started to bring together other Institutes and Government agencies to address this addiction. We want all conference participants to tell us what areas NIDA should be researching. This is vital information for NIDA to receive.

I also want to respond to an earlier comment about the common view of drug abuse as a problem affecting a small number of people rather than the larger population. When we speak to members of Congress about drug abuse, we find that they have this view of drug abuse. The points that have been discussed today about drug abuse as a disease and the changes that occur in the brain because of drug abuse may be useful in changing these views. Congress is concerned about the cost-effectiveness of drug treatment, and we have to convince them that a long-term perspective is needed. We need to show Congress something tangible and demonstrate that progress can be made.

Treatment

PSYCHOSOCIAL AND BEHAVIORAL TREATMENTS FOR WOMEN

Karla Moras, Ph.D.

Abstract

Few studies have examined the efficacy of different approaches to drug abuse treatment for women. Dr. Moras presented research findings about the efficacy of psychosocial and behavioral treatment strategies for drug abuse in general and for women in particular. Evidence suggests that women respond differently to the types of drug treatment used for men and that women may be more responsive than men to psychosocial and behavioral treatment. Interventions that emphasize increasing women's self-esteem and encourage choosing positive life options may be effective in treating drug abuse, particularly with adolescent females. Comprehensive treatment programs have been recommended widely, but their efficacy is still under evaluation. Dr. Moras cautioned that the term "female drug abusers" suggests that such women constitute a homogeneous group; however, in terms of treatment strategies, several subgroups must be studied: pregnant women (both adolescent and adult), injection drug users, adolescent polydrug abusers, older women, single professionals, and housewives.

Sex Differences in Drug Abuse Treatment Research

- There is little information about effective drug treatment strategies for women because women have been underrepresented in studies to date. The most widely quoted study of psychosocial treatments for opiate addiction, published in 1983, was conducted entirely with men at a Veterans' Administration hospital.

- Women are less likely than men to seek treatment for drug abuse, but women are more likely to seek treatment for psychiatric disorders and other medical problems.

- Some subtypes of female drug abusers may be more responsive than men to certain types of treatment. Psychosocial and behavioral treatments might be more effective with women than with men because of important differences in self-esteem and environmental and socialization factors, all of which influence maintenance of drug abuse behaviors.

- There is evidence that female drug abusers tend to have higher rates of comorbid mood and anxiety disorders than men who abuse drugs, and several studies have found that they also have lower self-esteem than men. Similar differences in levels of depression, anxiety, and low self-esteem also are found between women and men who are not drug users.

- Child-care responsibilities often interfere with women's ability to attend treatment programs.

- There are sex differences in employment options; women in drug abuse programs often lack marketable skills.

- The growing awareness of sex differences in treatment needs has led to a national focus on comprehensive treatment programs for female drug abusers. Comprehensive treatment programs currently are being implemented in many NIDA-funded demonstration grants, but data on their effectiveness are incomplete. These programs are aimed primarily at women who are chronic abusers of drugs such as heroin and cocaine, adolescents, pregnant women, and women who are poor or undereducated. Cognitive behavioral treatments for depression and anxiety may be useful to include in comprehensive treatment programs.

Conclusions From Literature Reviews

Dr. Moras presented conclusions based on literature reviews initiated by the NIDA Treatment Research Branch to determine the status of research on psychosocial and behavioral treatments for drug abuse.

- In most treatment studies, 50 percent or more of the eligible participants drop out early. Better strategies are needed to motivate people who abuse drugs to change their behavior patterns.

- Many people in drug treatment who achieve abstinence or significantly reduce their level of drug use often return to drug-abusing behaviors. This is true for treatment programs for all drugs, including nicotine.

- Psychosocial and behavioral treatments using contingency management techniques (such as a rewards system) are promising, but the behavioral change sometimes does not endure after the rewards cease. Research is needed on how to maintain behavior changes after the rewards stop.

- Many studies of psychosocial and behavioral treatments of drug abuse are flawed. For example, therapists may not be trained adequately to conduct the treatments being studied. However, methodological advances in psychotherapy research are being transmitted to the drug abuse field.

- Women, housewives, single female professionals, and older adults often suffer from overprescription of drugs. Education of practitioners about the appropriate approach to prescribing psychoactive medications for women is needed.

- Individuals who abuse hard drugs, such as heroin or cocaine, generally abuse more than one drug. For example, heroin addicts typically also abuse cocaine, and cocaine addicts also often abuse alcohol.

Issues for Future Research

- More research is needed on sex differences in the efficacy of psychosocial and behavioral drug treatment approaches and on treatments for women, including pregnant women. What psychosocial interventions are particularly effective in reducing some women's urge to take drugs?

- Self-esteem, life options, and environmental and socialization factors should be considered in the design of psychosocial treatments for women.

- More research is needed on ways to reduce drug-using behaviors and on methods to ensure that the behavior changes endure. Although contingency techniques have been found to reduce use of alternative drugs in methadone treatment programs (e.g., heroin-addicted people on methadone treatment who use cocaine as an alternative), individuals sometimes revert to drug-using behaviors when rewards are stopped.

- An important focus for future research is high-risk populations, such as adolescent females. Because studies of women who are chronic drug abusers show that identifiable behavior patterns appear during adolescence, targeting research on adolescents would be important to preventing drug abuse. Prevention interventions with adolescents should focus on improving life options and self-esteem.

- Research is needed on the overprescription of psychoactive drugs to women. Practitioners need to be educated about appropriate approaches to prescribing psychoactive medications for women.

- Comprehensive treatment programs are widely recommended; however, thorough trials, data analysis, and followup are needed to determine their effectiveness. The effectiveness of cognitive behavioral treatments for depression and anxiety should be examined more closely in such settings.

PHARMACOLOGY: SEX-SPECIFIC CONSIDERATIONS IN THE USE OF PSYCHOACTIVE MEDICATIONS
Sidney Schnoll, M.D., Ph.D.

Abstract

Studies of psychoactive drugs in nonhuman animals have found pharmacologic and pharmacodynamic differences between females and males, but the few studies conducted with humans have included only male subjects. High rates of anxiety and depression have been found among women who seek treatment for drug abuse problems, and studies show that women tend to seek medical help for emotional problems, whereas men tend to "medicate" themselves with alcohol and other drugs. Women are prescribed psychoactive medications nearly twice as often as men, but researchers have little information on the effects of these drugs on women, particularly when they are pregnant or of childbearing age. More research is needed on the effects of these drugs on women and the most appropriate treatment of psychiatric conditions.

Current Research on Psychoactive Drugs and Sex Differences

- Despite popular concern about overprescribing, most women are not being treated for the conditions diagnosed, although data indicate that psychiatric diagnoses are between 1.5 and 3.6 times more prevalent among women than among men. Furthermore, when women are treated for psychiatric diagnoses, they frequently are not treated appropriately. About 69 percent of patients diagnosed with major depression do not receive medication, even though antidepressant medication is effective. Women with anxiety syndromes are seldom treated with medication or given any other treatment.

- Most studies of psychoactive drugs are performed with laboratory animals, and there is evidence of pharmacologic and pharmacodynamic differences between male and female animals. Few human studies of psychoactive drugs are done, and most of those use young male medical students. Nonhuman animal studies do not indicate behavioral teratogenesis.

- Most drug companies do not study the effects of psychoactive drugs on women because of potential legal liabilities if there is danger of teratogenesis in subjects who become pregnant. Companies also avoid studies with women because menstrual cycles and hormonal changes may alter drug results. The menstrual cycle has dramatic effects on a woman's body, but research is rarely done on how psychoactive drugs affect the menstrual cycle. Studies of new drugs usually involve postmenopausal women.

- All psychoactive drugs are lipophilic (fat-soluble), and the differences in muscle mass and fat tissue distribution between men and women require that the drugs be administered differently. Also, the amount of time drugs are in the gastrointestinal tract is critical in drug absorption, and the transit time changes during the menstrual cycle.

- Many psychoactive drugs are not adequately studied among women of childbearing age, although these women have high rates of depression and anxiety and often are prescribed such drugs for treatment. The side effects of antipsychotic drugs occur more frequently in women than in men, so more care should be taken in prescribing these drugs to women.

- The placenta continually changes during pregnancy, and any drug that crosses the blood-brain barrier can pass through the placenta. The fetus is most at risk of adverse drug effects at days 18 to 55 of development. Most drugs have prolonged half-lives in the fetus, and therefore possible dysmorphic and behavioral teratogenicity are concerns. Most psychoactive drugs used during pregnancy, including antidepressants such as Prozac, produce a kind of neonatal withdrawal syndrome after delivery. Infants exposed to these drugs are often delivered prematurely and are undersized.

- There also are risks in not treating a pregnant woman for psychiatric conditions, including suicide, violence, and a decreased ability to function. If left untreated, the woman's physical and mental health may suffer, and she may refuse to accept prenatal care or abuse the fetus.

- Women are less responsive than men to imipramine in the treatment of depression, but the difference is not discussed in the literature. Older women metabolize benzodiazepines faster than men, and undesirable side effects from benzodiazepines occur more frequently in women.

Issues for Future Research

- Few studies examine sex differences in the effects of psychoactive drugs on humans. More research is needed on how drugs affect women of childbearing age, particularly pregnant women, and how women's hormones and menstrual cycles may influence the effects of psychoactive drugs.

- What is the appropriate method for treating depression and other psychiatric conditions in women, particularly pregnant women? Risks exist in both prescribing and not prescribing drugs to treat depression in pregnant women.

- Hard-core, long-term opiate addicts need a combination of psychotherapy, behavior modification, and pharmacotherapy. What combinations of behavioral therapies and pharmacotherapies provide the most effective treatment of anxiety, depression, and other psychiatric conditions for women in general and for drug-addicted women in particular? Practitioners typically give inadequate therapy, which can be worse than providing no treatment at all.

- Practitioners must be taught that cognitive behavioral treatments and antidepressants are highly effective and that proper prescribing of tranquilizers and pain medications reduces adverse effects.

RESEARCHER/SEX ISSUES
Jacqueline Wallen, Ph.D., M.S.W.

Abstract

Dr. Wallen addressed the issues and problems that researchers must consider when conducting studies of women who are in drug abuse treatment. Most drug abuse research has focused on men, and much of the recent research on women has been evaluation research focused on pregnancy-related areas. Research, including analysis of existing databases, is needed to determine (1) the characteristics of women in treatment for drug use, (2) the methods women use to finance treatment, (3) the pathways through which women enter treatment, (4) the kinds of services offered to and used by women, (5) the treatment outcomes for women in different kinds of programs, and (6) the costs and benefits of different treatment programs, particularly those that offer comprehensive services to women and their families.

Special Considerations for Research on
Drug Abuse Treatment Among Women

- Not enough data on women in drug abuse treatment have been collected and analyzed. NIDA and the Center for Substance Abuse Prevention have funded numerous demonstration programs for pregnant and postpartum women and their children. Some research findings have resulted, but there has been less research on women in drug treatment at other stages in the female life cycle. Characteristics such as low self-esteem, lack of child care, experiences of sexual abuse, and insufficient insurance may affect women's ability to enter drug treatment.

- The first step in collecting information about women is to find women with drug problems; their settings often are different from those of men.

- The Perinatal-20 study found that women who chose to enter treatment were less willing to accept random assignments in experimental studies. Such reluctance may present barriers to conducting research.

- Women are more likely than men to complete drug treatment, but a comparison of men and women in treatment who were at the same socioeconomic level found that women expressed more emotional distress. The assumption often has been that women experience more emotional distress than men, but Dr. Wallen suggested that men in drug treatment trials may not be expressing the emotional distress they actually feel.

Issues for Future Research

- There is commitment at the Federal, State, and local levels to make women's drug treatment programs comprehensive, but there is little research to support any particular drug treatment approach for women. More research is needed to determine the types of services offered to or received by women when they enter drug treatment. What are the costs and benefits, particularly of comprehensive programs? For which women are comprehensive programs most cost-effective? What are the treatment outcomes in different types of programs?

- It is important to determine the characteristics of women who do not enter treatment. What are the barriers for different groups? What factors facilitate the entry of women into drug treatment? Researchers should examine the large, national databases to identify the characteristics of women in drug treatment. Data are needed on income, health insurance coverage, age, marital status, sexual orientation, number and ages of children, race and ethnicity, housing situation, and primary language spoken. Type and severity of drug problems, psychiatric problems, history of sexual and other physical abuse, and HIV status are other factors that should be analyzed.

- It is important to conduct longitudinal research on infants and children regarding their resiliency and protective factors to help demonstrate the effectiveness of drug treatment in overcoming early risk factors.

- What are the characteristics of women who receive drug treatment from their personal physicians rather than from a treatment program? Do the treatment programs offer child care, medical care counseling, family planning services, HIV screening, parenting education, housing assistance, and transportation?

- How do women typically pay for drug abuse treatment? Which groups of women, and what proportion, pay for their own treatment, have private health insurance, or use community-sponsored drug treatment services? What are the costs of not treating women who need treatment—physical and mental health costs, protective services, income maintenance programs, and effects on families?

- What are the pathways through which women enter drug treatment? It is assumed that women are less likely than men to enter treatment via the correctional system, but there are conflicting research findings.

SERVICE PROVIDER/TREATMENT ACCESS ISSUES
Shirley D. Coletti, D.H.L.

Abstract

Dr. Coletti described Operation PAR, the largest nonprofit drug abuse program in Florida, whose programs feature innovative strategies to reduce barriers to drug treatment for women. Those innovations are important because few treatment programs focus on the special needs of women, the barriers they must overcome to obtain treatment, or ways to help women complete drug treatment. These barriers include (1) fear of separation from their children and lack of day care; (2) lack of safe, drug-free housing; (3) financial and legal difficulties; (4) health problems requiring services beyond drug treatment; (5) lack of knowledge about women and drug abuse; (6) lack of transportation; (7) long waiting lists for treatment; and (8) lack of youth-specific services. Because comprehensive drug treatment programs are expensive, collaboration among agencies is critical if such services are to be provided to women.

Barriers to Drug Treatment

- **Fear of separation from their children and lack of day care.**
  Many women leave treatment because they fear losing their children or being separated for an extended time. Some treatment programs ban communication between a woman and her family for 6 months. Operation PAR provides developmental day care for the children of mothers in drug treatment. Mothers can even participate in planning day care activities.

- **Lack of safe, drug-free housing.** Operation PAR overcame the housing problem in part by purchasing houses slated for demolition and moving them to its property.

- **Financial and legal difficulties.** Many female drug abusers are single parents with several children. Some women have a history of child abuse and neglect.

- **Serious health problems.** Women who abuse drugs often have other serious health problems. The trend toward HMOs or capitation plans may lead to a reduction in the number of health

58

care services provided to these women because such programs profit by providing fewer services.

- **Lack of knowledge about women and drug abuse.** Many health care professionals lack awareness and knowledge of some of the unique needs of drug-abusing women, particularly pregnant women. When physicians take medical histories, they often do not ask important questions that would enable them to diagnose drug addiction.

- **Lack of transportation.** Many women who abuse drugs have financial problems and rely on public transportation to see physicians or obtain treatment. Operation PAR provides transportation to clients with a fleet of about 30 vehicles funded in part by the U.S. Department of Transportation.

- **Long waiting lists.** Long waiting lists often discourage women who agree to enter treatment. Outpatient counseling encourages women to endure the wait for residential treatment.

- **Lack of youth-specific services.** Adolescents also need the full range of drug treatment services, but to be effective, services must be designed to meet the specific concerns of adolescents. Operation PAR has a 50-bed residential treatment program for female and male adolescents ages 13 to 17. It is a joint venture among the State of Florida, the county, private funders, and a bank.

DISCUSSION OF TREATMENT ISSUES

The discussion presented below dealt with treatment issues and followed the presentations of Drs. Moras, Schnoll, Wallen, and Coletti.

Dr. Christine Hartel: Are you aware of any governmental efforts to address problems you raised in testing drugs in pregnant women?

Dr. Schnoll: There has been a lot of effort in this area. Various government agencies now require the inclusion of women in testing programs. However, drug companies are concerned about liability issues and have not progressed very far.

Dr. Moras: What kind of incentives could be given to drug companies to study the effects of their agents on women?

Dr. Schnoll: The major issue is potential liability. Drug companies would be willing to do more tests on women if they did not have the risk of legal liability.

Dr. Mary Jeanne Kreek: The lack of studies among pregnant women is a critical issue. We did two studies on the pharmacokinetics of methadone given in steady doses to pregnant women who were not abusing other drugs. These studies were possible because one vendor was involved and provided pro bono services, and no pharmaceutical company was involved. Both my institutional review board (IRB) and the FDA agreed the studies were critical because they would lead to recommendations for the treatment of pregnant women. Only methadone and phenytoin have been rigorously studied. Do you know whether any additional drugs have been studied during human pregnancy with respect to pharmacokinetics?

Dr. Schnoll: Probably none have been studied. It is an appalling situation. My IRB demands that a drug prove efficacy in a nonpregnant population before it will consider a study in pregnant women.

Dr. Kreek: A prestigious university has insisted that pregnant women be included in a medications development study, but the medication has not been evaluated for teratogenicity. Investigators and IRBs need help in interpreting the guidelines for including women in studies and facilitating the development of needed studies that follow a step-by-step progression.

Dr. Schnoll: I agree. How do we start to develop studies on the interactions of behavioral therapies and pharmacotherapies? Such combinations may allow the use of fewer drugs and smaller doses.

Dr. Moras: Studies on depression show no evidence to support superior efficacy of combined drug and psychotherapy treatments. However, combined treatment would likely affect a higher proportion of people. Some will respond to the drug; some to psychotherapy. A colleague and I have requested a grant to study combined treatment for patients with drug-resistant depression. With comprehensive treatment programs for women, there is an underlying hypothesis that women more than men might benefit from combined psychosocial and drug treatment strategies.

Dr. Lisa Onken: NIDA is interested in encouraging research on the integration of behavioral and pharmacological treatments. A monograph on that topic will be coming out soon.

Dr. Karen Allen: As noted earlier by Dr. Moras, most treatments are not directed at housewives, single professionals, and older women. Do you have any recommendations for drug treatment for these groups?

Dr. Moras: One recommendation is educating health practitioners who serve those groups. A higher proportion of women than men present for treatment for panic disorder, and benzodiazapines are often prescribed, although there is evidence of a rebound effect when a patient withdraws. There is clear evidence that cognitive behavioral treatments are highly effective, as are some antidepressants. Perhaps educating health practitioners to stop overusing tranquilizers and overprescribing pain medications for women would be helpful.

Dr. Allen: What about treatment for alcohol, cocaine, and other drugs that housewives, single professionals, and older women sometimes use?

Dr. Schnoll: Part of the problem is that most practitioners are not trained to recognize drug problems in this population, and they do not take appropriate histories. With changes in health care delivery, primary care practitioners are going to be the gatekeepers. They must be trained to recognize the problems of addiction and how to treat it, mostly in their own clinical setting. Data indicate that 8 to 16 percent of a primary care physician's practice is composed of patients suffering from addiction, and most are not being treated for the addiction. Education is critical.

Dr. Dean Kilpatrick: Primary practitioners spend 8 to 10 minutes per patient. Training to screen and refer patients for drug treatment makes sense. Primary care practitioners who spend little time with each patient are not likely to be effective in treating such a complex problem as addiction.

Dr. Schnoll: We find that insurance companies are reluctant to pay for referrals to drug treatment programs; this is part of the move toward managed care.

Dr. Ruth Gordon: Some time ago there was an experiment to link mental health with primary care. Primary care physicians were trained, but there was no permanence because they did not do that kind of work continually. What can be done to support trained primary care physicians so that they continue to assess and treat people? What peer support can be provided?

Dr. Schnoll: There have been financial disincentives in the past associated with the kind of treatment and screening that primary care physicians should provide. With managed care, the financial incentives are there because the primary care physicians are responsible for the total health care costs and will seek to reduce their costs. Those working in drug abuse treatment need to offer more continuing education to primary care physicians.

Dr. Loretta Finnegan: I would like to see NIDA in a partnership with groups such as the American Society of Addiction Medicine to provide training to primary care practitioners, internists, and psychiatrists. Questions concerning addiction recognition and treatment should be included on medical boards. We must make the American Association of Medical Colleges aware that the prevalence of addiction is so high that it affects every other specialty. Medical students used to think they would not be dealing with addiction, but now they find that pediatricians have to care for babies undergoing drug withdrawal.

Dr. Joyce Roland: We are starting to address that issue. The North Carolina Governor's Institute sponsors a summer institute for health professionals at the University of North Carolina, and information about drug treatment is included. Is it possible to do animal studies in the lab that give an idea of how pregnant monkeys or rats might respond to certain medications? When we talk about how to approach pregnant women, what kind of work at the laboratory level is transferable?

Dr. Schnoll: If a drug company wants to use a drug with pregnant women, it has to do studies on several different species of animals to determine whether the drug is teratogenic. We have learned that a lot of information is not transferable—a drug may be teratogenic in certain animal species but not among humans and vice versa. It is difficult to do animal studies on behavioral teratogenesis.

Dr. Finnegan: Dr. Kreek, how much should a methadone dose be lowered when a woman wants to breastfeed?

Dr. Kreek: We conducted two studies on a small number of methadone-maintained patients who were not polydrug users and who had no serious medical or behavioral illnesses. Larger studies are needed. Earlier studies showed that less than 3 percent of orally administered methadone circulates in systemic blood, and less than 10 percent of methadone is free in plasma that can pass into breast milk. To be accurate, we need information on the volume of breast milk an average infant consumes after the first 2 to 4 weeks of life. With the information we had, we calculated that the amount of methadone that could pass from mother to baby was smaller than the dose of methadone a neonatologist would give a child for pain relief. Therefore, the amount of methadone delivered in breast milk is less than what an infant would have been exposed to in utero.

Although we do not hesitate to recommend breastfeeding to women on methadone maintenance[2] who have no other drug abuse problems, we do hesitate to recommend breastfeeding to women who have HIV. Of children born to HIV-positive mothers, 50 percent are HIV positive at birth. Of these, 20 to 35 percent are truly infected, but this cannot be determined until the child is at least 6 months old. If the child is not infected, an infected mother could expose the child to the virus through her breast milk. On the other hand, breastfeeding is good for babies from a psychological and immunological viewpoint. This is a difficult problem involving medical and ethical issues. We, in New York, hesitate to recommend breastfeeding for women who are infected with HIV.

Dr. Stephen Kandall: Based on Dr. Kreek's research, a local panel I chaired recommended that breastfeeding was acceptable and should be supported for methadone-maintained women who were not polydrug users and were not infected with HIV. However, the New York State Department of Health issued a document recommending that *all drug-using women* be discouraged from breastfeeding.[3] I do not know how that happened given the science that supports the safety of breastfeeding.

Dr. Kreek: I think we have to ask why scientific research information about drug abuse often is communicated inaccurately. Education is needed for physicians, nurses, social workers, and others to get rid of preconceived notions and bigotry about our patients. We know that hard-core, long-term opiate addicts need a combination of psychotherapy, behavior modification, and pharmacotherapy, but this knowledge still is not accepted.

Unidentified Audience Member: The FDA consent-to-treatment form for methadone maintenance also advises that these women should not breastfeed.

---

[2] Data are not available on the long-term effects of methadone in infancy.

[3] See footnote 2.

Dr. Marsha Rosenbaum: What effect does the combination of marijuana and methadone have in breastfeeding?

Dr. Kreek: I wish this question would be researched. I know of no study measuring levels of marijuana in breast milk. Another question is how much effect marijuana has on a person's behavior if it has been weeks since the drug was taken.

Dr. Schnoll: To answer that question would mean giving measured doses of marijuana to a woman who is breastfeeding and then getting samples of blood and breast milk. Such a study is not likely to be approved by an IRB.

Dr. Finnegan: Dr. Moras, you indicated that comprehensive care components include prenatal and neonatal care, family involvement, parenting skills, vocational training, employment counseling, medical services, and HIV risk prevention, and you said there are no data concerning these issues. Did you mean there are no data looking at all these components together? Do we have data on them separately?

Dr. Moras: Right, we do not have efficacy data on comprehensive multimodular programs.

Dr. Kandall: Given the effects of early influences on these women's lives, how likely is it that treatment will overcome those influences? How do we assess the effectiveness of treatment programs in terms of outcome variables?

Dr. Wallen: More longitudinal studies are needed on infants and children regarding their resiliency and protective factors, even though following a cohort of children for any period of time is expensive. This is extremely important research that should be done.

Unidentified Audience Member: Another issue being studied involves women who do not receive treatment services and those who are referred for drug treatment but refuse it. In addition, it is important to know the level of addiction a person has reached when she/he enters treatment because different levels produce different consequences and problems.

Dr. Rosenbaum: It is necessary to establish that there is common ground between researchers and research participants. In our experience, women can establish rapport with other women through one-on-one discussions. A major issue is how to help women access drug treatment if they cannot afford to pay for it. Lack of money to pay for treatment is a major barrier for some women.

Dr. Moras: One study reported that female drug abusers did not care whether those treating them were of the same ethnic or racial group; they were more concerned that those providing treatment services knew what they were doing and were helpful.

Dr. Peggy Stotts: Have researchers investigated how the attitudes of health care providers act as barriers to people in drug treatment? Bias on the part of providers has been recognized as a barrier because it discourages those seeking treatment.

Dr. Wallen: I agree. Some national databases collect data on facilities, their services, and whether staff members have had special training on women's issues. However, the data are collected at an aggregate level so there is no way to know how many women actually received services from providers who received the special training. We need more specific data about how services are delivered to those women who need them most. If you were making a recommendation for collecting national data, how would you suggest this question be asked?

Dr. Stotts: Health care providers should examine their own biases or attitudes toward women who use drugs during pregnancy and work through these issues so that they can provide nonjudgmental care to these clients. We need research to document the problem and address it through continuing education and medical schools.

Dr. Finnegan: We know that providers' attitudes toward men, women, and pregnant women can be very different. Addressing the problem requires more than a questionnaire. Nonverbal communication and interaction with clients can be observed by using videotape.

Dr. Kathleen Jordan: I have good news on this issue. At Research Triangle Institute, we are conducting two large, longitudinal, national studies of treatment clients. Your concerns about information gaps in research results are being addressed in some manner in these studies. One is DATOS, the Drug Abuse Treatment Outcome Study, which is funded by NIDA. The other is the National Treatment Improvement Evaluation Study (NTIES). Unfortunately, much of the funding for NTIES was used to support mainstream rather than enhanced services. I hope the studies that follow ours will learn from our experience.

Unidentified Audience Member: Early identification of women who are willing to enter treatment is important. Another important issue is the early development of children. A NIDA-funded grant that I am working on found that almost 50 percent of women in treatment neglected their children during the first 18 months and relied on the other family members for support. Are there studies of how to support the family while the mother is in treatment and incapable of caring for a child?

Dr. Wallen: I do not know of any such study. Very few of the large-scale databases collect information on whether women are ever offered financial or benefits counseling. It is important to know what support or benefits a treatment program can offer women so that barriers can be overcome.

Dr. Moras: I know of one model program that focuses on ways to involve the extended family of the pregnant or postpartum woman to provide help with parenting, as well as supporting her efforts to get off drugs.

Unidentified Audience Member: To get women into treatment, it is necessary to work with members of the extended family.

Etiology

THE ETIOLOGY AND GENETIC EPIDEMIOLOGY OF PSYCHIATRIC AND DRUG DISORDERS AMONG WOMEN

Kathleen R. Merikangas, Ph.D.

Abstract

Dr. Merikangas presented information about genetic epidemiology as a method of studying the gene-environment interactions that may be involved in the etiology of drug abuse. She described the appropriateness of applying the methods of genetic epidemiology to disorders such as drug abuse. She presented research data suggesting that drug abuse and drug dependence are transmitted in families and that sex is not a significant factor in the family transmission of drug dependence. Researchers found no distinct genetic factors underlying drug abuse in women and men.

Genetic Epidemiology Methods

Genetic epidemiology is the study of the etiology, distribution, and control of disease in families rather than in the general population. Unlike behavioral genetics, it focuses on diseases or disorders rather than traits and behavior patterns. Inheritance factors in genetic epidemiology refer to any factors that are transmitted in families, including cultural and biologic factors. Genetic epidemiology methods can be used to investigate whether sex differences in the prevalence of a particular drug abuse disorder are attributable to genetic or other transmissible factors.

In general, epidemiology ignores the family history of a disease or disorder even though it is one of the strongest risk factors for the etiology of chronic human disorders; instead, it provides information about the environment and the patterns of diseases in populations. Genetics focuses almost exclusively on host factors and fails to take into account the role of environmental influences. Therefore, researchers need to address gene-environment interactions when studying the genetic contributors to the etiology of drug abuse.

- One way to examine gene-environment interactions is to use study designs that control for the genetic background while letting the environment vary or vice versa. For example, the study of monozygotic twins (same genes) who are discordant for a particular disease is a powerful way to identify environmental factors that either potentiate or protect against the expression of the underlying genetic vulnerability.

- Twin offspring studies offer another approach. By controlling for family and genetic background (because the offspring of monozygotic twins are half-siblings rather than cousins), researchers can examine the role of factors such as exposure to peer networks, parents who abuse drugs, and parents with serious medical or psychiatric illnesses. Differences noted in these environmental factors help researchers identify factors that may lead to differential expressions in genetically similar individuals.

- The study of half-siblings who grow up in families in which the parents have divorced and remarried may help identify the role of drug exposure, environment, and family disruption.

- Studies of migrant populations may be the ideal way to identify the role of cultural influences on the development of a particular disease. Researchers can analyze changes in the disease rates of genetically similar groups who are from different areas of the world.

Research on Families and Risk Factors for Drug Abuse

- The National Comorbidity Survey showed that the rates of drug abuse and dependence are higher among males in the general population compared with females, a finding consistent with other epidemiologic studies across the United States. Therefore, the threshold for females to develop drug abuse is assumed to be higher than that for males. If females have a higher threshold for developing drug abuse, it is assumed that they would need to accumulate more risk factors, which then should cause greater rates of illness in both the male and female relatives of female probands. If genetic factors are responsible for the major sex differences in drug abuse and if women have more risk factors then men, then women's families should have greater familial transmission than men's.

- Data suggest that a family history of drug abuse is one of the most powerful risk factors for the development of drug abuse in individuals. Dr. Merikangas and colleagues recently completed a large, longitudinal family study (cosponsored by NIDA and NIAAA) of comorbidity of drug abuse, alcoholism, and anxiety disorders. Researchers from many disciplines, including psychologists, neurologists, sociologists, and anthropologists, interviewed children and other family members to determine what risk factors may be involved in the etiology of drug abuse.

- The study involved selecting a female proband and collecting family history information from parents, children, teachers, and other informants. Subjects were selected from both treatment settings and the community at large and were classified according to whether they had a major anxiety disorder, including panic disorder, social phobia, or agoraphobia. All probands met strict criteria for dependence rather than abuse of marijuana and anxiolytic drugs. A control group ("normals") selected from the community had none of the anxiety disorders and no history of drug abuse. Approximately 1,200 first-degree relatives and

250 spouses were interviewed. The researchers sought to understand the relationship among anxiety disorders, affective disorders, antisocial personalities, and drug abuse.

- The rate of drug dependence was 2 percent among relatives of the control group but was 12 percent among relatives of proband drug abusers. This suggested that there was a familial transmission or aggregation of drug dependence, and this transmission seemed to be specific to particular drugs rather than drugs in general.

- The nearly twofold increase in rates of drug dependence among male relatives confirmed the finding of population studies that men have higher rates of drug dependence than women. However, the sex of the proband made no significant difference in the drug dependence rates of relatives. When this hypothesis was tested in models that controlled for age, comorbidity, and other covariates, no sex difference was found in the transmission of drug dependence.

- After controlling for sex differences in base rates of psychopathology, no differences were found in the comorbidity patterns of male and female relatives, suggesting that comorbidity with affective and anxiety disorders in alcoholism does not lead to greater risk of drug dependence among relatives. After controlling for comorbid alcoholism in the probands, anxiety and affective disorders were not associated with an increased risk to the relative, suggesting some specificity in the transmission of drug abuse and the underlying etiologic factors.

- The data suggested that familial patterns of drug dependence were similar in families with relatives in drug treatment as well as in families from the community at large.

- Reports about drug dependence did not appear to be significantly influenced by whether the report was made by relatives or the individual proband. However, the information source was an important factor in reports about most psychiatric disorders.

Study Conclusions

- The data suggested that drug abuse and drug dependence were transmitted in families, but drug dependence appeared to have greater familial aggregation than abuse, particularly with respect to alcohol.

- There was specificity of transmission of drug abuse; that is, relatives of alcoholics who had no other drug abuse issues did not have elevated rates of drug abuse themselves, suggesting a difference in the etiologic factors for alcohol dependence and dependence on marijuana and anxiolytic drugs.

- After population base rates were controlled for, patterns of comorbidity did not differ between male and female drug abusers.

- Sex was not a significant factor in the transmission of drug dependence through the family. There were no distinct genetic factors underlying drug abuse in either men or women.

Issues for Future Research

- The key question over the next decade concerns the family characteristics that increase the risk of drug dependence and have a greater effect on dependence than sex differences. Research should be done on families with half-siblings to help identify the role of family disruption and environment in the etiology of drug abuse. Attempting to identify genes that increase the risk of drug dependence is too complex.

- The data suggested that drug abuse and drug dependence were transmitted within the family, but drug dependence appeared to have greater familial aggregation than abuse, particularly with respect to alcohol. To replicate and confirm these findings, a similar study of familial transmission of drug dependence is needed using individuals dependent on cocaine and opioids.

- What factors cause men to be at higher risk of drug abuse than women? Cultural and metabolic factors need further investigation.

- Research involving migrant populations is needed to identify the role of cultural influences on the development of drug disorders.

Questions From the Audience

The question-and-answer session below followed Dr. Merikangas' presentation.

Dr. Mary Jeanne Kreek: Did you use actual exclusion criteria for abuse or dependence of opiates and stimulants, including cocaine?

Dr. Merikangas: Many people were dependent on multiple substances so we looked at the relationship between alcohol and anxiety to see whether that extended to anxiolytic-type drug abuse. A person who had predominant cocaine dependence, opioid dependence, or any kind of injection drug dependence was not included in this study.

Dr. Kreek: Even the best instruments, such as the widely used Addiction Severity Index, do not measure magnitude of use and require only yes or no responses. Was the use of any of these drugs an exclusion criterion, or was it a question of what drugs were used predominantly?

Dr. Merikangas: Armed with the individuals' treatment records and detailed diagnostic interviews, we asked about drug preference, craving, and what the person would do if he or she had all the money in the world. We also looked at drug preference, duration of dependence on each substance, and age period when the individual used the substance. Based on this information, we tried to determine the major drug of abuse. For instance, if individuals had used cannabis, as most cocaine and opioid abusers do, from ages 13 to 14 and then never used it again, they would not be classified as cannabis users.

Dr. Kreek: This is important as we move toward more sophisticated molecular genetic studies, more sophisticated environmental risk factor impact studies, and their intersection. These data seem to show the dominance of other drugs over alcohol or, as you stated, a selectivity. Does that selectivity go even further within a drug group? It is difficult to judge how to label the phenotype in these kinds of studies. It will become critically important to include details about the instruments used and the cutoff criteria for those who used cannabis, anxiolytic drugs, or other substances. As far as outcome studies for the relatives, was the drug primarily one of the three that you named?

Dr. Merikangas: No. It could have been dependence on any drug. One of the major goals was examining specificity. We wanted to study not only the drug preference but also the specificity of actual drugs used among people who have been exposed to virtually every drug in their lifetimes. Many cannabis abusers have been exposed to a large number of different drugs, use cannabis daily, and have been doing so for 20 years.

Dr. Kreek: This is our finding, too, in the opiate-dependent group and more recently in the cocaine-dependent group. It is important in all the instruments to tease this information out and explain how it was done. Most studies still lump all drug abuse together, yet there are profound differences.

Dr. Brenda Miller: Please give more background on the characteristics of the proband group, particularly with regard to ethnicity, age, and social class.

Dr. Merikangas: With regard to socioeconomic class, all classes were represented. We also want to examine ethnic patterns to see whether there are differences in risk and drug use. Data presented today are for Caucasians only because the original study followed up on Dr. Myrna Weisman's family study of depression, which had an all-Caucasian sample. We extended the sample to include blacks and Hispanics. At present, we are analyzing some early data on blacks and Hispanics separately. The substance abusers tend to be in a somewhat lower social class than the control subjects. This is always a problem, but one that is controlled for in our analyses.

Dr. Miller: Many people assume the word "inherited" means genetic factors. I would encourage you to come up with a word other than inherited because the assumption is to equate that with genetics.

Dr. Merikangas: I agree with and appreciate your comment. Our work is designed to identify the noninherited factors and that is why I tend to use the term "transmissible."

Unidentified Audience Member: Were quality assurance procedures used by your interviewers? Was there a model that could be used by other programs?

Dr. Merikangas: Our priority was to have as interviewers clinicians who had clinical experience in asking questions about drug use and anxiety disorders. We used a diagnostic interview that is semistructured, so quality assurance was difficult. We have traded some reliability to gain clinical validity. Interviewers were trained carefully, using videotapes and group evaluations. Another clinician reviewed each interview that was done to ensure that the correct format was used. Periodically, someone observed each interviewer as she or he conducted interviews and performed a review of the interviewer's work.

Dr. Karen Allen: Is transmission of drug abuse through families more true for women than men?

Dr. Merikangas: No, the sex proband effect was not significant. Neither women nor men have a genetic vulnerability to drug dependence. Having relatives who abuse drugs increases a person's risk of having drug abuse by a factor of about 2.5. Knowing this helps to predict who may abuse drugs, but it tells us nothing about etiology. We need to understand what it is about the family that leads to drug dependence. We want to examine family background and explain why there is an increased risk of drug dependence and why some children in a family become dependent but their siblings do not. But this is just one study and requires replication.

Unidentified Audience Member: Why did you use semistructured interviews and focus on clinicians skilled in the disorders rather than use clinicians skilled in using the structured diagnostic interviews?

Dr. Merikangas: We were interested in psychopathology and its association with drug use. The structured interviews work well in obtaining information on drug and alcohol dependence. However, this is not true with regard to anxiety and affective disorders. The validity of some of the structured interviews was inadequate for examining the subtypes of anxiety and affective disorders. The so-called unstructured interviews actually were structured and coded, but the clinician made a "best-estimate diagnosis" based on more than the actual responses to the interview. Psychopathology—bipolar disorder, for instance—is usually missed by people who do not have some clinical experience or training in how to probe for relevant information.

Dr. Karla Moras: You can use clinically skilled diagnostic interviewers with structured interviews to reach the same goal. It is difficult for people who have no clinical experience to use a structured interview and obtain accurate diagnoses, but unstructured interviews are not a necessity. You have to hire skilled people.

Dr. Merikangas: Yes, particularly with children. The semistructured interview seems to be far superior in working with children.

Etiology Panel

CHILDHOOD AND ADOLESCENT PRECURSORS TO DRUG USE

Judith S. Brook, Ed.D.

Abstract

Dr. Brook presented data from a 20-year longitudinal study of precursors to drug use in children who were first assessed at 1 to 10 years of age and followed to young adulthood. Two main types of childhood personality attributes appeared to be important predictors of drug use during adulthood: (1) reckless and predelinquent behaviors, including aggression, and (2) poor emotional control. Specific predictors for drug use during childhood were associated with the development of personality attributes during early and late adolescence that, in turn, were related to higher stages of drug use in adulthood.

Longitudinal Study of Childhood and Adolescent Precursors to Drug Use

- A sample of 1,000 children, ages 1 to 10, was assessed in 1975. Investigators met with the mothers and the children, and both groups were reassessed during early and late adolescence. The last followup assessment occurred during young adulthood, when the subjects were 18 to 27 years old.

- During early adolescence, characteristics related to unconventionality were reported by young women who later had high stages of drug use: lower achievement, lower church attendance, greater rebelliousness, less responsibility, and greater tolerance of deviance. Those at higher stages of drug use reported difficulty in terms of emotional control (i.e., frequent expression of anger and impulsiveness). In the interpsychic area, only low ego integration was related to higher stages of drug use. Depression and anxiety were not related to higher stages of drug use.

- The behavior patterns of early adolescence persisted during late adolescence, although correlations were higher then, a result to be expected for predictions made closer in time to the present.

- The study findings supported using a mediational model to examine the relationship of childhood personality attributes to higher stages of drug use. That is, childhood personality risk traits were associated with the development of personality risk traits during early adolescence that related, in turn, to the development of personality risk traits in late adolescence. In turn, the risk traits of late adolescence were associated with higher stages of drug use in adulthood.

- Two main types of childhood personality attributes appeared to be important predictors of drug use during adulthood: reckless and predelinquent behaviors, including aggression, and poor emotional control, attributes similar to adolescent characteristics implicated in drug use. Early prevention efforts that focus on crucial personality attributes may not only inhibit initial drug use but also prevent drug use later in adulthood.

- Researchers identified several protective traits in childhood that can offset the effects of adolescent drug use on adult drug involvement over time, including achievement orientation during adolescence and a close mutual attachment between parent and child.

Followup Study Results

A followup study analyzed information on three generations over the 20-year study period: grandmothers, parents, and 2-year-old children. The analyses revealed the following:

- Drug use during adolescence and young adulthood appeared to interfere with the bonding relationship between these young women and their children. Personality attributes such as unconventional behavior, intrapsychic distress, or difficulty in relating to people also appeared to interfere with parent-child bonding. After controlling for personality traits, illicit drug use by parents directly affected the parent-child bonding relationship and reduced the expression of parental affection.

- There was evidence that illicit drug use by parents was related to poor social adjustment in the child. A history of unconventional behavior and intrapsychic distress in the parent strongly affected the 2-year-old's behavior; parents who were rebellious during adolescence and young adulthood had children who were not well adjusted socially and who expressed greater negativity and aggression.

- The risk factors for drug use in females at all developmental stages studied were found to be similar to those of males, but females exhibited lower levels of all the major risk factors. For example, females demonstrated lower levels of aggression, anger, predelinquent behavior, and hyperactivity and were better able to control their emotions and had friends who were not deviant and who were achievement oriented.

- One area in which females rated higher than males was intra-psychic distress, such as depression, anxiety, and obsessiveness. Intrapsychic factors are important in predicting drug dependence or abuse but not experimental or moderate drug use. Early and appropriate interventions can reduce risk factors for drug use among women and enhance protective factors.

Conclusion

Dr. Brook suggested that drug abuse prevention programs (1) focus on strengthening certain crucial personality traits that not only inhibit initial drug use but also may help prevent drug use during adulthood and (2) be initiated during childhood, because certain traits are precursors to adolescent drug use risk traits that later affect adult drug use.

Issues for Future Research

- A study similar to the research of Dr. Brook and colleagues is needed to examine childhood and adolescent precursors to drug abuse. A larger sample (more than 1,000 children) is needed to confirm whether illicit drug use by parents is related to increased negativity, aggression, and poor social adjustment in their children.

- Future research on sex differences should be based on a develop-mental perspective and include models that emphasize the interactive and reciprocal influences of the child, family, culture, and community. This broader approach will facilitate examining how different adaptive and maladaptive developmental pathways in females and males lead to drug use.

VICTIMIZATION AND POSTTRAUMATIC STRESS DISORDER

Dean G. Kilpatrick, Ph.D.

Abstract

Dr. Kilpatrick reported information from a retrospective and longitudinal survey of adult women in the United States that showed a clear relationship among assault, family history of drug use, posttraumatic stress disorder (PTSD), and sensation-seeking behaviors. Women subjected to violence had a higher risk of alcohol dependence and other drug abuse problems. Women who had alcohol or other drug problems, particularly with hard drugs, were at high risk of repeated assaults. PTSD is an important factor in alcohol and other drug abuse, and women often developed PTSD after experiencing a violent assault.

National Women's Study

Drug abuse disorders are more prevalent among women who have been crime victims. Several studies of drug abusers seeking treatment reveal that they have higher than average rates of past victimization. However, these studies seldom addressed the question of whether drug abuse occurred prior to violent assault or crime or whether the violent assault increased the risk of drug abuse. Is the relationship between violent assault and drug abuse a vicious cycle in which both events foster the development of the other?

Dr. Kilpatrick presented data from the NIDA-funded National Women's Study, a retrospective, longitudinal, national probability household survey of adult women in the United States. A random sample of women was interviewed by telephone. After the initial assessment, followup interviews were conducted at years 1 and 2. Complete followup information was obtained for 72 percent of the sample, and partial followup was accomplished for 83 percent of the sample. Aggravated assault was defined as an attack with or without a weapon but with the intent to kill or seriously injure the victim. New victimizations were defined as those that occurred during the followup interval. Current PTSD was measured by the National Women's Study PTSD module.

Initial Assessment—Wave 1

- It was found that 12.7 percent of the women surveyed had been victims of one or more completed rapes during their lifetimes, and about 10 percent had been victims of aggravated assault. Only about one in five cases of rape and aggravated assault had been perpetrated by strangers. Among women who had been assault or rape victims, more than half had experienced more than one type of criminal incident. Only 16 percent of rape cases and 46 percent of aggravated assault cases had been reported to police.

- The lifetime prevalence of PTSD was 12.3 percent; prevalence for the past 6 months was 4.6 percent.

- There appeared to be a linear relationship between the number of prior assaults experienced and the likelihood of lifetime alcohol dependence. Some women had experienced as many as three rapes or aggravated assaults prior to the initial assessment.

- The assessment also revealed other risk factors for the development of alcohol dependence: family history of drug abuse problems, high level of sensation-seeking, and lifetime history of PTSD.

- There was a clear relationship among assault, family history of drug abuse, PTSD, and sensation-seeking, even when the analysis controlled for other variables. Those who were alcohol dependent in the past were 25 times more likely than other subjects to be dependent on alcohol.

Followup Assessments at Years 1 and 2

Followup data at years 1 and 2 indicated a clear relationship between category of drug use at baseline assessment and an increase in the likelihood of suffering a new assault.

- About 28 percent of the sample used drugs, and a mutually exclusive grouping was used for analysis. A subgroup of polydrug or heavy drug abusers included those using heroin, cocaine, and any hard drugs or other substances. Another subgroup included those who used marijuana and alcohol but not "hard" drugs. Another subgroup included those who had met the *DSM-III-R* criteria for alcohol dependence and did not use other types of drugs.

- Of those women who did not use drugs at baseline assessment or may have used alcohol alone, 3.9 percent reported having experienced aggravated assaults during this period. Of those who met the diagnostic criteria for alcohol dependence, 6.1 percent reported having experienced new assaults. Even after controlling for past-year alcohol dependence, subjects who suffered a new assault were three times as likely to be alcohol dependent as other subjects. Of women who did not report any experiences of assault or rape at the initial assessment but experienced a rape or assault subsequent to that assessment, 16 percent developed an alcohol problem. After controlling for other variables, subjects with PTSD were found to be 5.5 times more likely to be alcohol dependent. Essentially, 100 percent of those women who experienced a prior assault or a prior alcohol problem and who developed PTSD also had an alcohol problem at followup.

- Of those who had used marijuana but not other drugs at baseline assessment, 9.6 percent had experienced new assaults. Of those who reported use of hard drugs at baseline assessment, 28 percent had experienced a rape or aggravated assault during the followup intervals.

- Among women who had ever received treatment for drug abuse problems (alcohol or other drugs), only 16 percent had no history of rape or aggravated assault and no PTSD. Eighty-four percent had experienced either an aggravated assault or rape or had developed PTSD. Forty percent had been assaulted but did not develop PTSD, and more than 30 percent of the group had experienced both assaults and PTSD. These figures are similar to data collected in other studies of women seeking drug treatment. Of particular concern is the young age at which most women who received treatment had been raped; 62 percent of the women reported being raped before age 18, and 30 percent before age 11. Other types of sexual assault were not included in these data.

Conclusions

- Women who have been subjected to violence have a higher risk of alcohol and other drug abuse problems.

- Women who have alcohol or other drug abuse problems, particularly with hard drugs, are at high risk of repeated assaults.

- Women who develop PTSD after experiencing an aggravated assault or rape are at greater risk of developing drug abuse problems. PTSD is an important factor in alcohol and drug abuse, and it is important to identify and address this disorder as soon as possible. Therefore, women in drug treatment programs should be screened to determine (1) whether they have been subjected to violent assaults in the past and (2) whether they have developed PTSD.

Issues for Future Research

- Future research should examine the presence of similar risk factors (e.g., alcohol dependence, PTSD, having been the victim of assault) in adolescents and young children; researchers found that most assaults were committed against adolescent girls before age 18.

- Clinical interventions designed specifically to prevent future assaults may increase clients' safety.

HARM REDUCTION

Marsha Rosenbaum, Ph.D.

Abstract

Dr. Rosenbaum stated that pragmatic treatment strategies are needed to help drug-abusing women who want treatment, particularly pregnant women. There is insufficient support for treatment programs, and most are not sensitive to the needs of women. Harm reduction is a viable strategy for minimizing the harm of drug abuse even if abstinence from drugs is not possible. She presented information from an ethnographic study that indicated that drug-abusing women who were pregnant used some form of harm reduction to achieve the best possible pregnancy outcomes given their drug abuse. More research is needed on these harm-reduction strategies and how to assist women with their efforts to minimize the harmful effects of drug abuse. Researchers and treatment specialists may have to accept strategies that minimize drug abuse and reduce its consequences rather than insisting on abstinence.

Findings on Harm-Reduction Strategies

Harm reduction is a pragmatic strategy that has been used in relation to methadone treatment for about 30 years and with AIDS patients who are drug abusers. Harm reduction emphasizes minimizing the harm brought about by drug abuse, even if drug abuse cannot be stopped completely.

Dr. Rosenbaum found that many women who abused drugs practiced personal harm-reduction strategies. The following findings are from a NIDA-funded ethnographic study of 120 women who were either pregnant or postpartum. The women used crack, heroin, or methamphetamine, and most were not in drug treatment.

- All women interviewed believed that their drug abuse would damage their fetuses and cause deformities, behavioral problems, or mental retardation. Reducing drug-related harm during pregnancy was imperative. The women varied greatly in terms of the harm they perceived and the strategies they used to reduce harm to their fetuses. Strategies included reducing or quitting drugs, attempting to counteract drug effects, improving diet, taking vitamins, getting more sleep, moving, changing lifestyles, and seeking prenatal care. Abortion was another method, but it was not a popular choice.

- Attempts to reduce drug-related harm seemed linked to the intensity of women's perceptions of possible harm. Crack users seemed to perceive their drug abuse as very harmful, which may be related to the large amount of media attention given to crack use. On the other hand, heroin users expressed less concern about drugs harming the fetus, which also may be related to the fact that stories about heroin and methamphetamine use appear in the news media less often than those about crack.

- Although all forms of drug treatment were considered by the women to be good methods for reducing drug abuse, drug treatment overall was not considered a sure solution. Many women combined drug treatment programs with their own methods of avoiding drugs. They were often not successful at permanently abstaining from drugs; temporary periods of drug abstinence were the norm. However, the women attempted to balance what they referred to as drug "cleanup times" with "mess-up times" and tried to maximize the cleanup periods.

- Another harm-reduction strategy was to combine or substitute the drug of choice with drugs that were perceived to be less harmful, such as replacing crack with marijuana.

- Health care services, particularly prenatal care, were perceived as the best way to improve health during pregnancy, but most women did not get as much health care as they wanted. They were more likely to disclose their drug abuse to health care providers during pregnancy so that they would obtain the best medical care possible, but they were likely to stop seeking health care during or immediately after pregnancy if they felt caregivers were judging them or ridiculing them for being pregnant and abusing drugs.

- In conclusion, data indicated that pregnant drug abusers often practiced harm reduction in some way.

Issues for Future Research

- More research is needed on how to assist women with harm reduction and the use of new strategies for harm reduction. How can treatment services be modified to complement the efforts of women to reduce the harm of drug abuse? Women who abuse drugs need more information about how drugs affect their health so that their efforts at harm reduction can be more successful. Dr. Rosenbaum asserted that women should have access to treatment even if they are not successful in being totally abstinent.

- Female drug abusers, particularly those who are pregnant, want and need health care services, but they will end contact with health care providers who appear to judge, blame, or humiliate them for their drug abuse. Drug treatment services should be designed to ease the problem of women avoiding or dropping out of drug treatment programs.

STRESS AND COPING AMONG WOMEN

R. Lorraine Collins, Ph.D.

Abstract

Dr. Collins presented the results of a survey on stress, coping, and drug use in a sample of nearly 2,000 female nurses in New York State. Prevalence of drug use among the nurses was compared with its prevalence among a subsample of women who participated in the 1991 National Household Survey on Drug Abuse (NHSDA). The key study question was whether stress and coping contributed to drug use or whether neuroticism influenced drug use. The definition of neuroticism included (1) anxiety and depression, (2) hostility, (3) self-consciousness, (4) impulsiveness, and (5) vulnerability. The nurses reported higher rates of prescription drug use than the women in the NHSDA. Cross-sectional analysis suggested that neuroticism was related directly to drinking alcohol as a way to cope with work stress and becoming acutely intoxicated but that it was not related to typical drinking. Future research should focus on longitudinal studies, studies of other populations, and examinations of sex differences.

Current Information From the Literature

Dr. Collins prefaced her findings with brief comments on what is known from the research literature on work stress and drug use, adaptive versus maladaptive coping, and the role of neuroticism.

- The existing literature is inconsistent as to whether stress and coping techniques are connected to drug use. There is little literature support for drug use as a direct response to work stress, but there is some support for the idea that job stress combined with ineffective coping strategies increases the potential for drug abuse.

- Drug abuse often is viewed as a short-term maladaptive coping strategy that provides temporary release from stress. Some literature suggests that women more often than men use maladaptive, or emotion-focused, coping strategies; therefore, it may be that women turn to drugs to alleviate anxiety, depression, and stress temporarily.

- Neuroticism has been linked independently to stress as well as to coping; therefore, it was hypothesized that it also may be linked to drug use. Highly neurotic people report more exposure to stress and appear to react more strongly to stress and to use maladaptive and ineffective coping strategies.

Findings of the Study on Stress and Drug Use Among Female Nurses

Dr. Collins presented information from a survey on drug use that was completed by 1,951 female nurses in the State of New York. Nurses were selected because their profession is highly stressful and allows easy access to medications, factors that are believed to place them at risk of drug abuse as a way of coping. The study examined the nurses' past and present use of alcohol, tobacco, caffeine, prescription drugs, and illicit drugs. The prevalence data from this survey were compared with data from the 1991 NHSDA on women in the northeastern United States.

- A high percentage of nurses reported using licit drugs at some time in their lives. Alcohol had been used by almost everyone, and there was a relatively high rate of caffeine and tobacco use. When these data were compared with NHSDA data, it was found that the nurses had higher rates of past-month and lifetime alcohol use. The rates of past-month tobacco use were approximately equal. (Caffeine use was not included in the NHSDA, and therefore data were not available for comparison.)

- The rate of prescription drug use, both past-month and lifetime, was higher among nurses than among women in the NHSDA, particularly for tranquilizers and barbiturates. This higher rate is a concern because health care professionals have easy access to drugs and are knowledgeable about their effects.

- The data on illicit drug use showed that the nurses used marijuana and opiates at higher rates but used cocaine at lower rates than the women in the NHSDA sample. The rate of hallucinogen use was about equal.

Subsample of Current Alcohol Drinkers

Data on a subsample of 637 nurses who were current alcohol drinkers were analyzed by causal modeling, and three alcohol-related outcomes were examined: (1) drinking to cope with stress at work, (2) typical drinking, and (3) drinking for the acute effects of intoxication.

- Data suggested that neuroticism led directly to alcohol-related outcomes; that is, drinking was used to cope with work stress. Data also suggested that neuroticism was related to the perception of stress, which, in turn, was related to alcohol-related outcomes. The data did not indicate any link between coping strategies and alcohol-related outcomes.

- Neuroticism was not related to typical drinking even though it was related to drinking to cope with work stress. This finding suggested that typical drinking was a response to social and cultural issues rather than a response to stress.

Future Research

Longitudinal studies are needed to determine whether there are causal relationships between neuroticism and drug use. Studies similar to those described by Dr. Collins are needed on drugs other than alcohol, and future study populations should be more heterogeneous and examine sex differences.

ETIOLOGY PANEL DISCUSSION

The discussion presented below followed presentations by members of the Etiology Panel: Drs. Brook, Kilpatrick, Rosenbaum, and Collins.

Unidentified Audience Member: We published an article in the *American Journal of Psychiatry* several years ago that analyzed data on the causal association and onset of drug abuse and PTSD. We did not collect data on incestuous rape, which usually occurs at young ages, so these events were not included in the analysis. However, our data from a sample of 3,000 people indicated that drug abuse preceded PTSD. We hypothesized that involvement in the drug culture put these people at risk for violent attacks and similar crimes. This is another area for future research.

Unidentified Audience Member: It is critical that we know more about childhood victimization before we assume which originates first: PTSD or other drug and alcohol problems. Data from a NIDA study of drug-abusing women indicate that childhood victimization occurs first, followed by signs of PTSD, and then by drug and alcohol problems.

Dr. Coryl Jones: Dr. Kilpatrick's study indicated that victimization often occurred before the age of 11, in children who were 6, 7, and 8 years of age.

Dr. Nan Vandenberg: First, what would be an ideal prevention program based on the strengths of these women that mediate the effect of drug abuse? Second, you noted that the young girls less likely to develop drug abuse disorders tended to conform to sexual stereotypes. Some research suggests that adherence to sexual stereotypes in adults can predict a greater potential for drug abuse. Can you explain this seemingly inverse finding?

Dr. Brook: For prevention programs, I would first focus on individual personality traits and include solid achievement-oriented activities. Second, some of our research showed that the atmosphere in the school is an important protective factor. Youngsters in a school where there was harmony among the administration, teachers, and students were more insulated from drug use. Youngsters in nondeviant peer groups benefited from that powerful protective factor, and finally, some aspects of the neighborhood and culture might be important. Researchers are just beginning to identify the protective and risk factors.

Consequences

MEDICAL AND HEALTH CONSEQUENCES OF HIV/AIDS AND DRUG ABUSE

Peter A. Selwyn, M.D., M.P.H.

Abstract

Dr. Selwyn gave an overview of the key issues of the HIV epidemic among women, with special reference to disease manifestations and clinical care. He pointed out areas of research relevant to the dynamics of this epidemic and presented epidemiologic information that suggested there were few sex differences in the progression of AIDS. Injection drug use is currently the most important risk factor for HIV infection among women. Recent studies indicate that HIV-infected women who use drugs are at higher risk of developing cervical abnormalities, gynecologic infections, and sexually transmitted diseases than HIV-infected women who do not use drugs. More research is needed on HIV infection among women and the medical and health consequences of drug abuse.

Overview of the Epidemiologic
Features of the AIDS Epidemic

- The rate of heterosexual transmission of AIDS has increased in the United States. In 1994 AIDS became the leading cause of death among young adult males and the fourth leading cause of death among young adult females. Among African-American women, it is the second leading cause of death, and in parts of the Northeast where AIDS is most concentrated among people of color, it has been the leading cause of death among both young men and women for several years.

- Injection drug use is the most important risk factor for HIV infection among women and accounts for half of all AIDS cases among women. One-third of AIDS cases among women have been attributed to heterosexual contact, and most involved contact with injection drug users.

Recent Research on HIV and Implications
for Improving Women's Health

- Drug abuse, particularly of cocaine, is one of several factors that seems to increase the risk for HIV infection. A 1991 study in New York found that crack use, prostitution, and sex in exchange for drugs predicted HIV infection among women, but a history of syphilis was not a significant predictor. Among men, syphilis was found to be a predictor, along with crack use and contact with prostitutes.

- A 4-year study in Louisiana found that HIV-positive women who injected drugs were at greater risk of developing sexually transmitted diseases than HIV-positive women who did not inject drugs.

- Studies have shown a strong relationship between cervical dysplasia and HIV infection. An Italian study of female drug abusers found that those infected with HIV were more likely than those who were not infected with HIV to experience cervical abnormalities, ulceration, and infection with common organisms.

- Dr. Selwyn suggested that, in addition to gynecologic disease, many differences in the manifestations of HIV/AIDS between men and women were primarily due to differences in screening, access to care, utilization of care, and stage of disease at presentation. An anonymous seroprevalence study found that, in an emergency room, male patients were more likely than female patients to be screened for HIV.

- Dr. Selwyn reported the results of several studies conducted at the Montefiore Medical Center with female and male drug abusers:

  1. There was high compliance among subjects when clinical care, including specific medical services for women, and methadone treatment were linked with AIDS research.

  2. No differences were found in the rate of progression to AIDS between the sexes or among racial and ethnic groups. There were no differences in AIDS progression because all subjects had equal access to care at the center.

- The overall manifestations of AIDS among women and men were similar after controlling for certain sociodemographic variables and gynecologic manifestations.

- No differences were observed between drug abusers and those who did not use drugs in terms of HIV progression. Dr. Selwyn believes the key to differences in disease progression was the lack of AZT therapy; drug use may be a barrier to AZT therapy.

- A study of a multicity, representative sample of HIV-infected people needing drug treatment services showed that up to half needed many other things such as mental health services, housing, home care, transportation, or entitlements. Dr. Selwyn noted that because many of these needs and circumstances affected outcomes, innovative approaches were needed to meet needs and improve outcomes.

- In a recent study of HIV transmission to infants in utero (ACTG 076), only 8.3 percent of the infants born to mothers who were treated with AZT during pregnancy were born infected with HIV, compared with 25.5 percent of those born to women who received a placebo. ACTG 076 is the first study to show a measurable effect of intervention in preventing HIV transmission from mothers to infants, and it raises significant issues that need scrutiny, such as how to identify women who may need AZT treatment and how best to counsel women and implement treatment.

- Several studies have found that among HIV-infected patients, women, drug abusers, and people of color are less likely than white men to be offered AZT treatment. Women who were injection drug users or had been incarcerated were much less likely to seek HIV care than women who had not used drugs or been in jail.

- Women who were drug dependent were found to be at high risk of violence and other abuse, but those who also were infected with HIV were at even greater risk.

Issues for Future Research

- Women with HIV infection are at risk of developing sexually transmitted diseases and other gynecologic problems. Research is needed on what diseases are specific to women with HIV and how they are manifested. Clinical manifestations specific to women need to be investigated thoroughly, including the efficacy of new HIV therapies.

- Much more research is needed on the etiology of HIV infection and finding methods to help women prevent infection at both the individual and community levels.

- More research is needed on eliminating barriers to health care for HIV-infected women and developing new models of care that integrate approaches from the biologic and social sciences. What are the most effective strategies for HIV screening and long-term followup? Are these strategies effective for women of color and poor women?

- Further research and more conclusive studies are needed on how to help women, particularly drug-abusing women, avoid common pathways to HIV infection. How can the rights of women be safeguarded in community programs designed to prevent HIV transmission?

- Research is needed on how best to identify women who are at high risk of HIV infection, particularly female drug abusers; how to make services available to them; how to consult with them before and during pregnancy about AZT intervention; and how to implement treatment that is effective and likely to have the desired outcomes.

Questions From the Audience

The questions and answers presented below followed Dr. Selwyn's presentation.

Unidentified Audience Member: Were patients in the clinical research setting offered any antiviral agents besides AZT?

Dr. Selwyn: At the time of the data collection, ddI (dideoxyinosine) was just becoming available through expanded access and compassionate-use programs. Since then, all the other antiviral agents have been offered through research, but women have shown little interest in most clinical trials. There is more acceptance of antiviral agents when they are prescribed by open label.

Unidentified Audience Member: What were the differences between women and men and active drug users and nondrug users regarding their willingness to comply with ongoing care that could detect the progression to AIDS?

Dr. Selwyn: In general, active drug use predicted nonadherence or worse outcomes in terms of followup for both men and women. However, other studies suggest that even active drug users outside a drug treatment program can be followed clinically in some areas and achieve relatively good treatment outcomes. It is unrealistic to conclude that a person using drugs cannot be treated effectively.

SOCIAL AND BEHAVIORAL CONSEQUENCES

Rafaela R. Robles, Ed.D.

Abstract

Dr. Robles gave an overview of research on drug abuse in Puerto Rico and compared data from a NIDA-funded study of AIDS among Puerto Rican and white women, conducted in both Puerto Rico and the United States. She noted a substantial increase in drug abuse among Puerto Rican women in recent years. Despite this trend, drug treatment programs in Puerto Rico and the United States have continued to plan and deliver services without considering the special needs of Puerto Rican women. Dr. Robles asserted that there is an urgent need to integrate social support services with nonpunitive drug treatment services for women. Drug treatment programs must be based on an understanding of the ideology, sociocultural perspective, and needs of Puerto Rican women and their families. Puerto Rico is one of the epicenters of the AIDS epidemic, and drug addiction is the primary risk factor for both men and women.

Trends in Drug Abuse in Puerto Rico

- Dr. Robles and her colleagues assessed the drug abuse education needs of health care personnel in Puerto Rico and found that nursing and medical education curriculums had little instruction on drug abuse except for pharmacology-related information. The clinicians surveyed wanted more information on drug addiction and legal and policy issues, especially those related to women.

- There has been a substantial increase in drug abuse among Puerto Rican women. More women than men seem to be abusing barbiturates, sedatives, tranquilizers, and amphetamines. A survey of high school adolescents found that more girls than boys were smoking. More women than men are becoming HIV-infected through drug abuse or having sex with drug abusers. Female sex workers who abuse drugs are more likely to be HIV-positive than their peers who do not abuse drugs.

- Despite these trends, many health and drug treatment centers in the United States and Puerto Rico continue to deliver services without considering the special needs of women, and in Puerto Rico, most do not recognize and address drug abuse among women unless it is related to motherhood.

- In Puerto Rico, women are seldom offered HIV testing in settings other than family planning clinics. Late recognition of HIV infection and poor access to services may contribute to the different patterns of disease progression and survival in women and men.

- Sociocultural biases are reflected in legal actions against drug-abusing mothers. Such actions include the removal of newborns from their mothers and court-ordered detentions of pregnant women who abuse drugs. Women of color and low-income women are disproportionately affected by punitive legal measures, and fear of such actions discourages women from obtaining drug treatment and social services.

Early Findings of an AIDS Demonstration Research Study

- Dr. Robles presented the early findings of the NIDA AIDS Demonstration Research Project among Puerto Ricans. The data were drawn from 996 female subjects who abused drugs: 351 islanders (those residing in Puerto Rico) and 287 Puerto Ricans and 358 non-Hispanic whites living in the United States.

- Both groups of Puerto Rican women were more likely than whites to live on welfare. Puerto Rican women living in the United States were most likely to use illicit methods to obtain money. Most Puerto Ricans in the United States (77.4 percent) were unemployed, followed by whites (65.9 percent), and islanders (49.9 percent).

- Drug-abusing women in Puerto Rico had a high HIV seroprevalence rate (41.6 percent), similar to that of drug-abusing men. Logistic regression analysis showed that a history of incarceration, injection drug use for more than 6 years, lack of condom use, and syphilis were significantly associated with HIV infection. Women ages 25 to 34 were at highest risk.

- People who were HIV-positive tended to use more safe sex measures than those who were not HIV-positive. The reasons behind this finding are unknown.

Research on Sex Differences Among Drug Abusers in Puerto Rico

- A comparison of drug-abusing men and women in Puerto Rico found that more women than men had completed high school, lived with their children, and received support from the government. Women were more likely to engage in oral and anal sex, have multiple sex partners, and trade sex for money. They were more likely to use health services.

- Puerto Rican drug abusers who had social support reported fewer psychiatric symptoms and physical illnesses and were more likely to live longer than those who had little or no social support. Women were more likely than men to live with their children in their own homes and to have conflict with family members. Men were more likely than women to rely on family members for support, especially with regard to completing drug treatment. However, drug-abusing women, those both in and not in treatment, were more likely than men to report feeling depressed and attempting suicide, a finding that is consistent with previous studies in the United States.

- There were large differences between women and men in experiences of physical abuse. Nearly one-third of the women reported having been physically abused during childhood, and 21 percent said that they had been abused in the previous year.

Issues for Future Research

- Research is needed on which drug treatment programs and services are most effective in meeting the needs of Puerto Rican women who abuse drugs. What are the differences between women who receive treatment and those who do not?

- More research is needed on the effect of social policies and laws on people who abuse drugs, particularly women. Are low-income women or women of color disproportionately affected by legal actions, such as the removal of newborns or court-ordered detention of those who are pregnant? How do such policies affect their willingness to enter drug treatment?

Consequences Panel

THE CONSEQUENCES OF DRUG DEPENDENCE ON SOCIAL SUPPORTS, HIGH-RISK SEXUAL BEHAVIORS, AND HOMELESSNESS

Adeline Nyamathi, R.N., Ph.D.

Abstract

There has been insufficient research on the psychosocial predictors of risk behaviors and coping behaviors of women, in terms of both AIDS and drug addiction. Knowledge of these risk factors and their influence may suggest effective new strategies for intervention programs. Dr. Nyamathi presented information from a 5-year study of factors that predicted risk behavior in African-American and Latino women who resided in homeless shelters and in residences provided by drug recovery programs. A Comprehensive Health-Seeking and Coping Model was used to examine situational, personal, and sociodemographic factors; community resources; cognitive appraisal; threat appraisal or perception; coping skills for managing threats; and outcome variables. Self-esteem was found to be an important predictor that affected all other variables, including social support, emotional distress, threat appraisal or perception, barriers to condom use, active coping and avoidant coping skills, drug abuse, and AIDS and sexual risk behaviors. It is important to implement culturally sensitive intervention strategies that will enhance women's coping skills, self-esteem, and social support. More research is needed on the psychosocial predictors of both risk behaviors and coping behaviors related to drug abuse among women.

Five-Year Intervention Study of Risk Factors Among Women in Poverty or Drug Treatment

Previous research has shown that women with high self-esteem or social support are less likely to perceive threats in their environment, more likely to cope adaptively with problems, and less likely to experience emotional distress. Dr. Nyamathi's study hypothesized that women with greater self-esteem and social support were likely to experience little emotional distress, perceive fewer threats in their environment, and experience fewer barriers to condom use. Therefore, they also would be likely to use more active coping techniques, engage in fewer AIDS risk behaviors, and use drugs less often.

The researchers further speculated that individuals with greater emotional distress were likely to perceive more threats, experience more barriers to condom use, use more avoidant coping techniques, engage in more AIDS risk behaviors, and abuse drugs more often. They hypothesized that coping was associated with risk behaviors and that ethnicity and acculturation were related to all of the other psychosocial variables.

The subjects included 714 African-American women and 691 Latino women who were recruited from drug recovery programs and homeless shelters. Nurses and outreach workers of African-American and Latino backgrounds administered the survey questionnaires, and the content and semantics were examined to ensure that they were valid and culturally appropriate.

Self-esteem, social resources, and emotional distress were defined as predictor variables; threat perception, barriers to condom use, and coping were considered mediating variables. AIDS, sexual risk behaviors, and drug abuse behaviors were defined as outcome variables. Drug abuse behavior was measured in terms of noninjection drug use, injection drug use, and sharing needles.

The women in the study were separated into three groups for data analysis: African-Americans, highly acculturated (HA) Latinas, and less acculturated (LA) Latinas. Many of the hypothesized relationships were supported by the models.

- Fifty-nine percent of African-American women used non-injection drugs, compared with 25 percent of HA Latinas and 4 percent of LA Latinas. Injection drug use was highest among HA Latinas (23 percent), compared with African-American women (10 percent) and LA Latinas (1 percent).

- Self-esteem was an important variable and affected all the others. Among African-American women, self-esteem was positively related to a high level of social resources and negatively related to emotional distress. The higher the social supports, the higher the self-esteem and the lower the emotional distress. The relationships among the variables were similar among African-American and Latino women, except that for Latino women, self-esteem was not related directly to barriers to condom use.

- Emotional distress was the main predictor of threat perception. Individuals with more distress tended to use avoidant coping and were more likely to use drugs. Dr. Nyamathi speculated that interventions that reduce emotional distress may influence women's perceptions of threats. A high level of threat perception predicted barriers to condom use for both African-American and Latino women. In addition, a high level of threat perception combined with avoidant coping predicted drug abuse. Active coping indicated less AIDS risk and drug abuse behaviors; therefore, enhanced coping skills are critical to drug abuse intervention strategies.

- Among Latinos, social support predicted barriers to condom use, and AIDS and sexual risk behaviors among Latino women were predicted by barriers to condom use, threat perception, and avoidant coping techniques. The higher the acculturation level, the greater the barriers to condom use and the greater the level of AIDS, sexual risk behaviors, and drug abuse behaviors. Interventions with Latino women need to incorporate elements of the traditional Latino family and community to strengthen support for condom use.

Conclusion

The cross-sectional design of the study limited the conclusions that could be made about causal relationships, but it is clearly important to implement culturally sensitive intervention strategies for women that will enhance coping skills, self-esteem, and social support. This research begins to pinpoint the ways in which personal resources influence healthy behaviors.

Issues for Future Research

- More research is needed to assess the psychosocial predictors of drug abuse and AIDS risk or sexual risk behaviors among women who live in poverty. Research also is needed to test models for assessing the psychosocial predictors of health-seeking and coping behaviors among poor women.
- The differences in psychosocial predictors among racial and ethnic minority groups need to be identified so that culturally appropriate interventions can be designed, developed, and evaluated.

PSYCHIATRIC SEQUELAE OF DRUG ABUSE
Linda B. Cottler, Ph.D.

Abstract

Dr. Cottler's presentation focused on the psychiatric sequelae of drug abuse in women, such as antisocial behavior and depression. She stressed the importance of researching psychiatric issues related to drug abuse because these topics often receive little attention. There are differences between women and men in the psychiatric sequelae of drug abuse, but such differences also can be found among subgroups of drug-abusing women in terms of age, socioeconomic status, and other factors. Data were examined on early drug abusers (those who started drug use by 15.7 years of age) and later drug abusers (those who started drug use by 18.8 years of age). Early drug use was associated with greater drug abuse and phobic, depressive, and antisocial disorders. These findings point to the need for more studies to develop effective strategies for treating psychiatric disorders in women who abuse drugs.

Results From Two Studies

Dr. Cottler merged data on drug abusers from two studies conducted in St. Louis. The two samples included people who had received drug treatment and those who had not been treated but had consented to be in the study. The data on women were stratified to identify patterns, such as age of initial use and the use of cannabinoids, amphetamines, sedatives, cocaine, heroin, opioids, PCP, hallucinogens, and inhalants. The results were as follows:

- Early drug abusers (those who started drug use by 15.7 years of age) were more likely to be alcoholics than later drug abusers (those who started drug use by 18.8 years of age).

- When data from the St. Louis studies on antisocial personality (ASP) disorder and subtypes were examined, some women met the criteria for ASP disorder but had not been formally diagnosed. Later drug problems seemed to be associated with later antisocial adult behavior. Early drug abuse by women was characterized by more irritable and aggressive behaviors, such as repeated physical fighting and physical attacks on partners. Early drug abusers also showed less remorse for hurting people or stealing than did later drug abusers.

- Almost all early drug abusers had used cannabis, and 60 percent had used amphetamines, compared with 27 percent of later abusers. Early abusers tended to use multiple drugs, including cannabis, amphetamines, sedatives, and cocaine, and 68 percent used injection drugs. Later drug abusers used primarily cannabis and cocaine. However, the two groups did not differ significantly in terms of being diagnosed with drug abuse or dependence, except that early abusers were more likely to be alcoholics. The earliest symptom of drug abuse or dependence was hazardous drug use or use with increased risk of injury, and this symptom appeared when the women were about 20.2 years of age.

- Other research has found that externalizing disorders, such as ASP disorder and other personality disorders, are more common among men than among women, whereas internalizing disorders are more common among women. Data show that women may be subtyped in terms of psychiatric sequelae and that psychiatric diagnoses are much more prevalent among drug-abusing women than they are among women in general.

- Drug abuse begins at about the same time as antisocial behaviors, but depression starts after the onset of drug abuse and may be a consequence of drug abuse. About 30 percent of the St. Louis research participants had attempted suicide, and 54 percent had thought about dying or committing suicide.

Issues for Future Research

- Research is needed on the psychiatric conditions found in different subgroups of women who abuse drugs, such as those of different ages and those who use different types of drugs. It is important that comorbid psychiatric conditions be assessed and that levels of drug addiction be analyzed.

- Research is also needed on antisocial and depressive behaviors among drug-abusing women, both singly and in combination, because women are more likely to seek treatment for depression than for antisocial behaviors. Studies are needed to develop effective treatment strategies for women.

Questions From the Audience

The question-and-answer session presented below followed Dr. Cottler's presentation, which was part of the Consequences Panel.

Unidentified Audience Member: There is controversy about whether certain people who are diagnosed with ASP disorder really should receive that diagnosis on the basis of drug abuse-related behaviors. With regard to ASP rates among the women in the study, particularly those who had only adult symptoms, have you looked at the issue of how many of the behaviors labeled as antisocial are a direct result of the drug abuse as opposed to being a distinct antisocial type?

Dr. Cottler: The old criteria for an ASP diagnosis eliminated anything caused by other drugs and alcohol, and this restricted the prevalence rate of drug abuse somewhat. But we found that some researchers mark the responses they get in the drug section. For example, if someone is an injection drug user, that is automatically counted toward both drug use and the antisocial behavior criteria. We did not do that in our study.

Unidentified Audience Member: What about other behaviors that are directly the result of drug abuse but are not actual drug abuse? For example, the only time someone steals is to get money for drugs. Have you tried to look at that factor when you separate the actual effects of the drug abuse from other types of antisocial behaviors?

Dr. Cottler: That is a good point, but it is extremely difficult to ask respondents to tell you why they stole money—whether it was because of drugs or something else. But this is an important issue for people who do this kind of research to figure out when they are asking questions and doing the algorithms for antisocial behavior.

PARTNER VIOLENCE

Brenda A. Miller, Ph.D.

Abstract

Dr. Miller discussed recent research on partner violence and its relationship to drug abuse. Research shows that women who abuse drugs regularly and are in drug treatment programs are significantly more likely to report partner violence than women in the same treatment settings who do not abuse drugs regularly. Preliminary data from a NIDA study showed that 90 percent of women in drug treatment had experienced severe violence from a partner during their lifetimes. Women from the general population in the same geographic area who were not in drug treatment had a significantly lower rate of violent experiences. The data indicate that drug treatment interventions are important in addressing partner violence and its effect on women's treatment outcomes. More research is needed to determine whether there is a causal relationship between drug abuse and partner violence.

Earlier Studies on Family and Partner Violence

Data have indicated a connection between partner violence and drinking among both women and men. However, most violent situations occurred when neither partner had been drinking; therefore, drinking is not a necessary correlate of partner violence.

The analysis of national data has revealed that the combination of blue-collar occupational status, drinking, and the approval of violence is closely associated with high levels of violence.

NIAAA Study of Women in New York State

Dr. Miller reported the results of a study sponsored by the National Institute on Alcohol Abuse and Alcoholism (NIAAA) of 472 women in western New York. The women were from outpatient alcoholism clinics, classes for alcohol-impaired driving, battered women shelters, outpatient mental health clinics, and the general population.

There was a significant difference in the amount of severe partner-to-woman violence among women in alcoholism treatment compared with women in the general population. Women who regularly abused drugs and were in treatment (treatment for alcoholism, mental health outpatient services, or battered women's shelter) were significantly more likely to report partner violence than women in the same treatment settings who did not regularly abuse drugs. Although women in the sample may have had several partners during the course of the study, these findings endured regardless of which partners were involved.

Preliminary Data From NIDA Study of Women in Drug Treatment

Dr. Miller presented preliminary data from a NIDA study examining drug issues and drug problems among two groups of women in the same geographic area; one group was in drug treatment, and the other was not. A third group of women was recruited from battered women shelters and matched with a group of women who were not in shelters but who lived in the same geographic area.

- Preliminary data for the women in drug treatment and the matching general population sample showed that 90 percent of women in drug treatment had experienced severe violence from a partner during their lifetimes. The rate of severe partner violence in the general population sample was high, but it was significantly lower than that experienced by women in drug treatment, even after the women had been in drug treatment for 6 months.

- There were no significant differences in rates of violence between the women in the two groups selected from the general population, but there were significant differences in the rates of partner violence when the women in drug treatment and in shelters were compared with the women in the general population groups.

- It is not known whether partner violence is a consequence of drug abuse or vice versa. Dr. Miller noted that the NIAAA study found a slightly stronger connection for victimization experiences predicting alcohol problems than the reverse; therefore, the possibility of a connection exists. She speculated that acute intoxication or chronic abuse of alcohol or other drugs may make a person vulnerable to victimization; however, she cautioned against blaming drug abusers for being the victims of violence.

Implications for Drug Treatment and Prevention

- It is important that drug treatment strategies for women address partner violence and its implications for treatment outcomes. Support systems for women need to be designed to respond to the problems of partner violence and alcohol and other drug problems. Most shelters and drug treatment settings address only one of the two problems.

- Dr. Miller asserted that there is an acceptance of violence in our society that is an environmental and social barrier to drug treatment and needs to be addressed. Treatment or intervention strategies that focus solely on individual change are ineffective if the drug abuser must return to the same environment and stresses encountered before entering drug treatment.

Issues for Future Research

- Is partner violence a consequence of drug use or vice versa? Does victimization make women more vulnerable to alcohol and other drug problems? What is the relationship between partner violence and drug abuse? How does partner violence affect a woman's treatment outcome? Treatment programs for drug abuse must take into account the significance of violence and the woman's history of victimization.

- Researchers who seek to develop more effective drug abuse interventions for women must recognize and examine the intergenerational patterns of family violence and alcohol and other drug problems. Individual and cultural differences need to be recognized.

- Researchers need more time to analyze data and write and disseminate their research findings so that myths about drug abuse are not perpetuated. Better methods are needed to disseminate research findings and ensure their application in the health care system.

Questions From the Audience

The discussion points presented below followed Dr. Miller's presentation, which was part of the Consequences Panel.

Dr. Judith Brook: There is a possibility that drugs and victimization may eventually demonstrate a reciprocal model. Assuming that drug use has a later impact on victimization, two important mechanisms to explore are the family and types of friendships or social networks. It also might be useful to control for some personality traits because it is known that they are related to alcohol and other drug use and may be related to victimization as well.

Dr. Miller: I think you have two good points.

Prevention

LINKS BETWEEN PREVENTION AND TREATMENT
Karol L. Kumpfer, Ph.D.

Abstract

Dr. Kumpfer presented information from the research literature on the links between drug abuse prevention and treatment among drug-abusing women and their families. She noted the need to design drug abuse prevention programs that focus on specific research-based risk factors, such as poor maternal-child relationships, child abuse and neglect, sexual abuse, partner violence, posttraumatic stress disorder, poverty, and the excessive stress and social isolation often experienced by single parents. Drug treatment programs that strengthen the family and include parent training, family therapy, and children's skills training successfully reduce children's interest in drugs. Little research has been done on drug abuse prevention for women and adolescents who do not have children, and programs for high-risk female adolescents are rare.

Current Information on Drug Abuse Prevention and Children

There is little research on drug abuse prevention for women and adolescents, although there is mounting research on drug abuse risk factors. Most current information is based on research conducted with the children of alcohol-abusing parents, but recently research has been conducted with the children of parents who abuse drugs other than alcohol to identify similarities.

- Research has shown that children of drug abusers are at high risk of future drug abuse. They use drugs at higher rates than children in the general population, but drug treatment programs for women rarely address preventing their children's drug abuse. Early research findings suggest that the children of drug-abusing parents can develop resilience that makes them less vulnerable to stress.

- Five years of research on drug treatment and prevention have indicated that the behavioral and emotional problems of children are reduced in a relatively short time when mothers are trained in parenting and family skills, including therapeutic child play. These changes also reduce the mother's level of drug use and stress.

- Researchers have found that a variety of environmental and biological factors may increase a child's risk of becoming a drug abuser. Environmental factors that contribute to drug abuse include poor family relationships and communication; increased conflict; poor discipline style characterized by inconsistency, repressiveness, or violence; lack of adult supervision and unrealistically high expectations of children; sexual or other physical abuse of children; parental and sibling modeling of drug use; mental or physical illness; criminal involvement; and poor school environment.

- Child neglect and abuse are significant factors predicting drug abuse; studies have shown that about 19 percent of opiate-abusing families and 27 percent of alcohol-abusing families had children who were neglected to some degree.

Results of the Strengthening Families Program

Dr. Kumpfer described the results of the Strengthening Families Program (SFP), a family skills training and drug treatment demonstration program funded by NIDA that includes 14 weeks of parent training, family therapy, and children's skills training.

- Drug-abusing parents and their children benefited from participation in an intensive program in which a counselor role-modeled desired parent-child interactions with parent and child, observed the parent-child interaction, and then reinforced improved behaviors. Skills training and family therapy were an important part of the drug treatment process for mothers. Randomized clinical trials funded by NIDA suggest that SFP helped the mothers become better parents, increased their self-esteem, and reduced their depression.

- Children in the program had less interest in starting to use drugs, and those who already used drugs began to reduce their level of use. There were significant decreases in the children's level of aggression, depression, conduct disorders, and social withdrawal.

These results have been replicated in other studies, and the results have been robust in programs that were modified for different racial and ethnic groups and in those conducted in both urban and rural communities.

**Recommendations for Drug Abuse Prevention
Among Women and Children**

- Women at high risk need to be recruited into prevention programs, and drug-abusing women need to be recruited into treatment programs. Recruitment is difficult, but the most successful programs are those that develop a trusting environment and provide child care, transportation, and social services.

- Prevention programs need to educate mothers about birth control and about the consequences of their drug abuse on their children. Programs should be based on specific, research-based risk factors in mothers: poor maternal-child relationships, child abuse and neglect, sexual abuse, partner violence, posttraumatic stress disorder, poverty, and the excessive stress and social isolation experienced by single parents.

- Drug abuse prevention efforts with adolescent girls should focus on preventing school dropout and increasing academic success; preventing pregnancy, sexual abuse, and eating disorders; enhancing mother-daughter relationships; teaching social skills, particularly in choosing friends and boyfriends; and conducting parent-peer support groups in the school.

- Treating the total family unit is critical to any lasting improvement in the family system. Unfortunately, most women's drug treatment programs do not do this, despite research on the psychology of women that suggests women's relationships to children and significant others are critical to mental health. It is necessary to intervene in the multigenerational process of dysfunctional families and drug addiction. Children should be taught life skills to help them develop resilience and cope with drug-addicted parents.

Issues for Future Research

- Research is needed on sex-specific drug abuse prevention efforts. Drug abuse treatment professionals and researchers need to work together to ensure that etiological research results are translated into effective drug abuse prevention programs for women and their children. Research is needed on prevention and treatment efforts with women and adolescent girls who do not have children; most previous research has focused on those who have children.

- More research is needed on the parent-child relationship and why the children of drug-abusing parents are more vulnerable to drug abuse. Is it due to in utero exposure, parental drug abuse, or poor parenting? What are the differences between children of alcohol-abusing parents and those whose parents abuse other drugs? Are there differences in terms of genetics, environment, in utero exposure, or direct versus passive exposure? Prevention programs that focus on children from birth to age 6 need to be developed.

- Early research suggests that children who live with drug-abusing parents may have increased competencies and resilience to stress because of the challenges and stresses they are inadvertently exposed to. More study is needed on what can be done to strengthen the resilience of these children.

- Programs for adolescent girls should focus on school dropout prevention, academic encouragement, sexual abuse prevention, mother-daughter relationship enhancement, eating disorder prevention, and assistance with social skills such as choosing friends and boyfriends. What are the factors that cause some adolescent girls to lose interest in academic success as they mature physically? Parent-peer support groups also are needed.

Questions From the Audience

The question-and-answer session presented below followed Dr. Kumpfer's presentation.

Dr. Risa Goldstein: Have you or anyone else applied the "Strengthening the Families" interventions in residential treatment settings?

Dr. Kumpfer: These interventions have been used in methadone maintenance programs and mental health outpatient clinics. Although they are appropriate for residential programs, they require additional staff training. A residential program that already involves children presents an ideal opportunity for a demonstration program.

Dr. Judith Brook: Your program seemed to be developmentally appropriate, taking into consideration the age, stage of development, and sex of the child.

Dr. Kumpfer: Our program is for 6- to 12-year-olds. We desperately need a program for children from birth to age 6 because these are the ages of most children who are in residential programs.

Dr. Brenda Miller: We tend to overlook teenagers when we develop drug abuse prevention programs, but the teenage years are when drug use patterns are established. Could you comment about where we might go in prevention programs for teenagers?

Dr. Kumpfer: We have not seen the prevention field move toward programs for adolescent females. We need to work with these adolescents on the importance of academic success and how to choose good friends. Peer influence is a most important factor in their risk for becoming drug abusers. It is important to help parents understand and communicate with their teenage children.

Dr. Miller: The teenagers who most often have problems with drugs and early pregnancy are those who are estranged from their parents. Some families do not believe they need to protect their teenage children. When you hear about a teenage girl's sexual activity, it is always assumed that the activity was her choice. Our models for prevention do not address the complexities of that age group.

Dr. Kumpfer: You have raised an issue that could be addressed, for example, through harm-reduction programs to help girls avoid date rape or sexual abuse. Such programs would be useful for younger girls as well as for girls in junior high and high school. It is also a good idea to reach parents, perhaps through public service announcements, and remind them that they need to protect their children.

Intervention

INTERVENTION, OUTREACH, AND SPECIAL NEEDS

Kathy Sanders-Phillips, Ph.D.

Abstract

Dr. Sanders-Phillips addressed the correlates of health behavior among low-income women from racial and ethnic minority groups and the implications for drug abuse prevention and intervention. Drug abuse is a health or risk behavior that represents the endpoint of a series of health decisions. Dr. Sanders-Phillips' research indicated that there were highly significant ethnic differences, not only in the health behaviors of black and Latino women but also in other related factors. In almost every category, Latino women were more likely than black women to engage in healthy lifestyles and behaviors. Dr. Sanders-Phillips suggested examining the roles of internalized racism and exposure to violence to determine what effect they have on drug abuse among women from racial and ethnic minority groups. The study findings reaffirmed the conclusion that the social and cultural environment has a substantial effect on the health behaviors of these populations.

Information From the Research Literature

- Research at the University of Pittsburgh indicates that life events, physical health problems, and internalized racism have an important effect on alcohol abuse by black women. Religious orientation has an inverse relationship with alcohol consumption and is correlated positively with internalized racism in black women.

- Physical health problems and internalized racism are significant predictors of depression among black women. Dr. Sanders-Phillips asserted that the data raise the possibility that factors such as internalized racism may mediate the relationship between depression and drug abuse.

- There is evidence that exposure to daily violence creates feelings of powerlessness, hopelessness, and alienation that influence women's health behaviors, decisions about family planning and prenatal care, and relationships with their children.

Study of Health Promotion Behaviors and Barriers

Dr. Sanders-Phillips asserted that by examining drug abuse in the larger context of women's health decisions and behaviors, it is possible to identify the correlates of drug abuse and health behaviors and identify factors that increase the risk of drug abuse. She recruited 243 black and Latino women from Head Start programs in south-central Los Angeles for a study that examined how frequently women engaged in four health behaviors: eating breakfast, sleeping 7 or 8 hours per night, exercising at least three times per week, and using alcohol or tobacco. This research confirmed the importance of social and cultural factors in women's health behaviors and decisionmaking.

- Race and ethnicity were significant factors that predicted health promotion behaviors. In almost every category, Latino women were much more likely than black women to engage in healthy lifestyles and behaviors. Only 21 percent of black women ranked health as a first priority in their lives, compared with almost 51 percent of Latino women. More black women than Latino women ranked religion as their first life priority. The data suggest that social and ecological factors are significant correlates of health behaviors.

- Health behaviors, with the exception of exercise, were correlated highly with low consumption of alcohol and other drugs. Women who reported eating breakfast and sleeping 7 to 8 hours per night tended to report lower levels of alcohol and tobacco abuse.

- A woman's perception of the health care worker and whether the person truly cared about her health was another important factor in whether she engaged in health promotion behaviors.

- Black women were more likely than Latino women to report good or excellent health status, and they were much more likely than Latino women to be employed and to have health insurance. Latino women were more likely than black women to perceive their health status as fair or poor.

- Black women were more likely than Latino women to report experiences of violence. Exposure to violence was negatively related to engaging in healthy behaviors. The findings suggest that exposure to violence, perhaps in addition to direct victimization, may influence health behaviors, including alcohol and other drug abuse.

Issues for Future Research

- More studies are needed to examine the racial and ethnic differences in the factors associated with the health behaviors and correlates of drug abuse among women. Is there a relationship between internalized racism and health behaviors? Research on internalized racism may provide information about sources of stress for women from different racial and ethnic minority groups and will help develop more effective intervention programs.

- It should be determined whether exposure to violence increases the abuse of illicit drugs or serves as a precursor to individual victimization. Are there racial and ethnic differences in the relationship of exposure to violence and victimization to health behaviors and drug abuse?

Questions From the Audience

The questions and answers presented below followed the presentation by Dr. Sanders-Phillips.

Dr. Rafaela Robles: Are there studies that have used acculturation as a mediator variable? Migrants who are not integrated into mainstream society often do not know how to use the health care system.

Dr. Sanders-Phillips: We looked at acculturation, but we were dealing with a sample that was not highly acculturated. Some literature suggests that as Latino women become more acculturated, their health behaviors become poorer. These findings have tremendous implications for our understanding of drug abuse in that population.

Dr. Robles: With regard to the finding that Latino women's health behaviors worsen as they become acculturated, it has been said that Americans do not like to acknowledge being sick because they do not want to miss work. Another important variable is migration status. Recent migrants often are not integrated into the health care system because they have not become acculturated.

Dr. Sanders-Phillips: The main message is that for researchers to understand the health behavior patterns of different groups, they have to examine the social experiences of those groups.

Dr. Robles: When I compare data on drug abuse among women in Puerto Rico and Puerto Ricans living in the United States, I find large differences because of the differences in the social experiences between those groups. For example, in Puerto Rico, we are not a minority as we are in the continental United States.

Dr. Sanders-Phillips: I believe that minority status and social experiences are tied to Taylor's finding of relationships between internalized racism and health behavior.

Dr. Nan Vandenberg: Taylor's study has suggested that within the gay and lesbian population, the use of drugs is 20 to 30 percent.

However, most researchers ask subjects about marital status rather than sexual orientation, and therefore, homosexuality often is not identified. If 20 to 30 percent of the gay and lesbian population are drug addicted, it may be explained by internalized homophobia in confluence with sexism and racism. I think we need more studies that examine sociocultural contexts.

If Latino women were more likely to engage in healthy behaviors, why did they feel less healthy?

Dr. Sanders-Phillips: That question has intrigued me, and we are still investigating it. Rates of depression tend to be high among Latino women, and the literature suggests that they may somaticize this depression. My data also suggest that many of Latino women's health habits are culturally determined so they may not be making conscious decisions about their health behaviors.

Unidentified Audience Member: Black women in the study said they were slightly more likely to exercise than Latino women. Why was this not reflected in their overall health behaviors and lifestyles?

Dr. Sanders-Phillips: That is another intriguing question. Exercise was correlated less highly with other health behaviors, and evidence in the literature suggests that other health behaviors are influenced more by psychological factors such as stress and depression. But exercise patterns are also affected by stress and depression, so psychological factors are one potential answer. The ethnic difference is related in part to the perceptions of danger in the community, which were higher among black women.

Dr. Joyce Roland: Do you have a method or an instrument that measures internalized racism?

Dr. Sanders-Phillips: Jerome Taylor at the University of Pittsburgh has a scale to measure internalized racism.

Dr. Roland: A factor contributing to the finding that black women feel more healthy than indicated by their health behaviors might be their belief that God will take care of them.

Dr. Sanders-Phillips: I believe the discrepancy between perceptions of health status and health behavior is explained in part by possible ethnic differences in how women define health status and related factors. I believe there is a historical precedent, particularly for black women in this country, to define oneself as healthy because health is related to the ability to take care of one's family, but this ability may be unrelated to how a person feels.

Unidentified Audience Member: Did you control for the fact that Mexican-Americans, in the Southwest in particular, are so eager to please that they often give positive answers, which can bias the questionnaire results? Also, did immigration status affect whether they had insurance coverage? A third question is whether you identified their religious affiliation, because the Catholic church has a significant influence on the Latino population. Were the concepts of alternative medicine and the use of shamans and healers that are popular among Mexican-Americans considered in the findings?

Dr. Sanders-Phillips: We did not look at alternative therapies, but we are aware of their use. We avoided direct questions about immigration status because they tend to create fear that mitigates against the trust we need. We recruited, to the extent possible, through the Head Start program and had the support of teachers in the classroom. This increased the probability that we would get more truthful answers from the Latino women. Also, the questionnaires were in Spanish and were administered by Spanish-speaking interviewers. It was easier to recruit Latino women possibly because they are eager to integrate into the mainstream system. Black women, for the most part, have given up on that hope.

Unidentified Audience Member: Latinos tend to be predominantly Catholic. How does internalized racism relate to the religious message?

Dr. Sanders-Phillips: We did not look at that, but I would say that there are implications in the broader system. However, an investigator who has examined power differentials between physicians and patients from racial and ethnic minority groups found that the greater the power differential, or the perception of it, the less likely women were to engage in healthy behaviors.

Dr. Judith Brook: Our research shows that there are a number of risk factors that are similar in different racial and ethnic groups. A study in East Harlem found some major differences between African-Americans and Puerto Ricans in terms of protective factors. For example, among African-Americans, modeling was important in terms of family, mentors, and the general environment. Among Puerto Ricans, behavioral modeling had more to do with the dynamics of the family interaction.

Dr. Sanders-Phillips: We need to examine the racial and ethnic similarities as well as the differences. But we should not confuse the fact that there may be similarities in risk factors with the possibility that there may be differences in the situations and environments that cause those risk factors. Similar risk factors may be associated with different experiences in different groups of women.

Legal and Criminal Justice Issues

PUNISHING WOMEN FOR THEIR BEHAVIOR DURING PREGNANCY: AN APPROACH THAT UNDERMINES THE HEALTH OF WOMEN AND CHILDREN

Lynn M. Paltrow, J.D.

Abstract

Ms. Paltrow provided an overview of the issue of civil and criminal punishment as applied to drug-abusing pregnant women, with special emphasis on its negative effects. She also presented some suggestions, as formulated by the Coalition on Alcohol and Drug Dependent Women and their Children, for avoiding the adverse affects caused by such legal actions.

Background

For more than a decade, Government officials have sought to punish women for drug-using behavior during pregnancy. Some advocates of "fetal rights" argue that children should be able to sue their mothers for "prenatal injuries."

Women's and children's advocates agree that women should engage in behaviors that promote the birth of healthy children, but they recognize that a woman's drug abuse involves complex factors that must be addressed in a constructive manner. Punitive approaches fail to resolve addiction problems and can undermine the health and well-being of women and their children. For this reason, public health groups and medical organizations uniformly oppose measures that treat pregnant women who abuse drugs as criminals.

Many types of prenatal conduct can harm a fetus or cause physical or mental abnormalities in a newborn, including smoking, drinking alcohol, failure to obtain prenatal care or proper nutrition, environmental hazards, and the contraction of or treatment for certain diseases, such as diabetes and cancer. Charging mothers with the crime of child abuse according to the health or condition of the newborn child would subject many mothers to criminal liability for engaging in all sorts of legal or illegal activities during pregnancy.

Criminal Prosecution

Although no State has enacted a law that specifically criminalizes prenatal conduct, prosecutors have used child abuse and neglect statutes to charge women for actions that potentially harm the fetus. At least 200 women in more than 30 States have been arrested and criminally charged for their alleged drug use or other actions during pregnancy.

All appellate courts reviewing criminal charges and guilty verdicts based on a woman's prenatal conduct have ruled that criminal statutes must be strictly construed in favor of defendants, and words such as "child" may not include the fetus. Courts have unanimously held that drug delivery laws apply solely to circumstances in which drugs are transferred between two persons already born. Courts also have refused to apply murder or feticide statutes in such cases, concluding that those laws were never intended to punish a woman for prenatal conduct affecting her fetus or to hold her criminally liable for the outcome of her pregnancy.[4]

Negative Effects of Punitive Laws

Punitive measures can be counterproductive by causing pregnant women who are drug abusers to avoid prenatal or medical care for fear of being detected and severing them from the health care system, thereby

---

[4] In July 1996 the Supreme Court of South Carolina became the first appellate court in the United States to uphold a prosecution of a woman for child abuse based on her use of a drug during pregnancy. In a divided 3-to-2 opinion, the court ruled that a viable fetus is a person for the purposes of South Carolina's child neglect law and that a woman could be prosecuted for any behavior that poses a risk of harm to the viable fetus and be subjected to up to 10 years in prison. A petition for rehearing is pending in this case.

increasing the potential harm to both mother and fetus. Although only a minority of States have laws that mandate reporting to civil child welfare authorities in cases where a newborn is dependent on or tests positive for an illicit drug, hundreds, if not thousands, of women across the country have had their children taken away because of a single positive drug test.

In numerous States, legislators have introduced measures that would provide prosecutors and courts with explicit authorization to penalize pregnant and parenting women with drug abuse problems. To date, no State has expanded its criminal code to punish women who are pregnant and use drugs, although approximately 10 States have revised their civil child protection laws to require the reporting of a newborn's positive drug test.

Legislative Efforts

The failure to pass any criminal statutes and the limited adoption of the mother's prenatal drug use as evidence of civil child neglect reflects, in part, the overwhelming opposition by the medical community and its recognition of the extreme shortage of drug treatment programs for pregnant women.

Recommendations

The Coalition on Alcohol and Drug Dependent Women and Their Children recommends the following legislative action to improve maternal and child health:

- Provide that pregnant women may not be subjected to arrest, commitment, confinement, incarceration, or other detention solely for the protection, benefit, or welfare of her fetus or because of her prenatal behavior. Any person aggrieved by a violation of such a provision should be allowed to maintain an action for damages.
- Provide that positive toxicology tests performed at birth may be used only for medical intervention and not for the child's removal without additional information being obtained on parental unfitness, which assesses the entire home environment.

- Provide that child abuse reporting laws may not be triggered solely on the basis of alcohol or other drug use or addiction without reason to believe that the child is at risk of harm because of parental unfitness.

- Provide that alcohol and other drug treatment programs may not exclude pregnant women and increase appropriations for comprehensive alcohol and other drug treatment programs.

- Utilize existing funds for the prevention and treatment of alcoholism and other drug dependence among women and their families.

- Review agency services and propose the coordination of related programs among alcohol and other drug treatment programs, social services, education, and the maternal health and child care field to improve maternal and child health.

Questions From the Audience

The discussion presented below followed Ms. Paltrow's presentation.

Dr. Kathleen Jordan: The majority of women in North Carolina prisons have high rates of drug abuse and other psychiatric disorders. Most have been victimized from early childhood, abused by family members, thrown out of their homes, and involved with male partners who abused drugs and were abusive. Prisons present an opportunity to provide drug abuse treatment to many women who have demonstrated motivation to change their lives.

Ms. Paltrow: The female prison population has tripled since the war on drugs began. Women in prison are denied many things; neither pregnant women who give birth while in prison nor other mothers can see their children. On the one hand, we need treatment in prison. On the other hand, if better services are available in prison than in the community, it could send the message that a woman has to be convicted of a crime to get help.

Dr. Loretta Finnegan: Thank you for suggesting communication among Government agencies. NIDA's divisions communicate with other agencies; for example, NIDA has an interagency agreement with the Center for Substance Abuse Treatment and the Administration for Children, Youth, and Families.

Ms. Paltrow: When you are a public figure, it is hard to have any cause of action for libel. Sometimes it is possible to get a correction from the media, which can be more effective than the original report. Perhaps the solution is more speech and more correction rather than silencing or punishing the media.

Dr. Coryl Jones: NIDA is active with the Federal Interagency Panel on Child Abuse and Neglect, which brings together the Departments of Defense, Justice, Health and Human Services, and Agriculture—all the programs that work with children and families in the United States and in the military abroad.

Unidentified Audience Member: Please address how the probation system affects women, particularly women who abuse drugs.

Ms. Paltrow: In many legal cases, woman are poorly advised and plead guilty to nonexistent crimes. Some feel that probation is a way to avoid having to deal with the courts. However, if they relapse to drug use, and without treatment they are likely to relapse, they will end up in jail.

Crosscutting Issues Panel

AFRICAN-AMERICAN WOMEN AND TRAUMA: DEPRESSION, DRUGS, AND FAMILIES

Sheryl Brissett-Chapman, Ed.D., A.C.S.W., L.I.C.S.W.

Abstract

Dr. Brissett-Chapman asserted that the analytical approach to understanding African-American women and drug abuse poses serious cultural constraints. For African-American women, trauma is represented more by the chronic and unmitigated life circumstances they face than by a series of assaults or events. Research efforts and methodology that take a more comprehensive and synthesizing approach are needed. Applying scientific observations to the qualitative experiences of African-American women who abuse drugs will help produce more effective treatment programs. African-American women who abuse drugs need structured settings in which building self-esteem, self-responsibility, and parenting education is combined with drug treatment. In addition, the development of extended family support systems is critical to helping these women after they leave drug treatment.

Depression

- Depression among African-American women is an adaptive, coping response to their traumatic life circumstances and the perception that they have few options in life. For African-American women, trauma is caused more by chronic and unmitigated life problems than by assault. The stigma associated with being homeless, abusing drugs, or failing to care adequately for one's children has a powerful effect on African-American women and contributes to their depression.

- African-American women who abuse drugs, are homeless, or are in prison have to develop survival skills to cope with the trauma in their lives. Reliance on these skills has become normalized for many women in shelters and prisons. Dr. Brissett-Chapman asserted that this normalization of survival skills has serious implications because it leads to social alienation, family violence and victimization, abandonment, unmet personal needs, and, most important, unresolved grief and loss issues.

Drug Abuse and Families

- Eighty percent of the residents of the Baptist Home for Children and Families are African-American women. Although they do not come to the shelter for drug treatment, 40 to 50 percent have drug abuse problems. Other factors that compel women to enter the shelter include unresolved childhood sexual abuse, evictions, overcrowding, job loss, and lack of job skills.

- Women often must leave their homes to escape violence by their partners, which also may involve sexual abuse of children; 30 to 40 percent of the women at the shelter have problems with domestic violence. In 95 percent of domestic violence cases, the male perpetrator abuses drugs.

- Drug abuse by family and friends is a problem for many of the women because they may not be able to limit these relationships and their effects and because they do not have alternatives for housing and support.

Recommendations

- Structured, supportive programs are needed to help African-American women confront drug abuse, depression, and family problems. Successful treatment programs include components such as self-esteem support groups and interagency planning. At the Baptist Home for Children and Families, women work with the staff to develop a plan for their families' futures. An extended family system is important to help them deal with depression and avoid drug abuse. Such support should include help for depression, treatment incentives, recognition of needs, and a redefined sense of community and family. Parenting education is critical because it increases mothers' self-esteem and their hopes for their children. They need to experience incremental successes in various aspects of their lives to support their efforts to stop drug abuse.

- Women in drug treatment need to be supported until they are ready to go to permanent housing or other arrangements. Most treatment programs are too short and unforgiving of drug relapse, and traditional 12-step programs usually are not sufficient for these women. At the Baptist Home for Children and Families, the average stay is 5 months. During this time the women must take care of their children, follow curfews, assume responsibilities, comply with drug treatment (although relapses are seen as part of the path to recovery), and try to meet self-determined case management goals.

Issues for Future Research

- The analytical model cannot be applied to African-American women because it poses serious cultural constraints. Research is needed to identify the qualitative experiences of African-American women and to combine this information with analytical research so that more effective drug abuse treatment programs can be developed.

- More research is needed on the identity and psychological development of young African-American females and their vulnerability to developing depression and abusing drugs to cope with traumatic life circumstances. How can the needs of African-American women be recognized, and what incentives will help them confront depression and avoid drugs?

- Research is needed on how to address the need of many drug-abusing African-American women for external support and extended family systems. How can a new sense of family and community involvement be encouraged?

DRUG ABUSE AND HIV AMONG LESBIANS
Marjorie J. Plumb, M.N.A.

Abstract

Ms. Plumb identified shortcomings in research conducted on drug abuse and HIV among lesbians, including a lack of data on sexual orientation among general population surveys. The stigma that society associates with lesbians has hindered progress on research in this community. Some studies have found that some subpopulations of women who have sex with women, such as IV drug users, are at higher risk of HIV infection than comparable subpopulations of heterosexual females. Ms. Plumb suggested that lesbian researchers be consulted on how to design and conduct research studies on drug abuse in this population.

Current Knowledge

Ms. Plumb asserted that there are three major problems with the drug abuse research that has been conducted in the lesbian and gay communities:

1. Research on HIV, AIDS, and drug abuse often does not include gathering information on lesbians because researchers assume that all their female subjects are heterosexual. It is difficult to adequately conduct research on drug abuse behaviors among lesbians because many women believe that identifying themselves as lesbians may put them at risk of losing their children, jobs, or housing.

2. Many lesbians accept only specific terms to identify their sexual orientation, and different terms can confound researchers. For example, some women who have sex with women do not identify

120

themselves as lesbian or bisexual. In addition, an individual's sexual identity and behavior can change over time.

3. The lesbian community is reluctant to deal openly with drug abuse and HIV issues because society already stigmatizes these women for their sexual orientation. Some treatment providers reportedly advise lesbians not to discuss their sexual orientation while in treatment to avoid homophobic situations and treatment personnel who inappropriately pathologize lesbianism.

Ms. Plumb presented the following observations from research that has been conducted with lesbians:

- One study suggested that more lesbians than heterosexual women smoke cigarettes and that lesbians consume more alcohol for longer periods. Other studies found that lesbians use alcohol in combination with other drugs more often than women who responded to the 1990 National Household Survey on Drug Abuse. The National AIDS Demonstration Research Projects found that women who had sex with women were more likely than heterosexual women to use drugs and be homeless. Research in 1994 indicated that 23.5 percent of lesbians ages 26 to 34 had used marijuana in the preceding month, in contrast to 9.1 percent of women of the same ages in the 1990 National Household Survey on Drug Abuse.

- Lesbians are at higher risk for HIV infection than heterosexual women, who are otherwise demographically similar. A Seattle study of women entering a drug treatment program found lesbians to be five times more likely to be HIV-positive than other women. In a 1993 seroprevalence study in San Francisco, 1.2 percent of lesbians were infected with HIV, a rate three times higher than the estimated rate of HIV infection among all women and adolescent girls. From this random sample of lesbians and bisexual women, 10.4 percent reported using injection drugs since 1978, with 3.8 percent reporting injection drug use during the preceding 3 years. Seventy-one percent reported sharing needles, and 31 percent reported sharing needles with gay and bisexual men.

- The Centers for Disease Control and Prevention (CDC) reports that about 1 percent of women with AIDS are lesbians (CDC defines lesbians as women who have had sex only with women since 1978). But Ms. Plumb observed that this definition may exclude a large number of women, and the data are incomplete, possibly because of the heterosexist bias of providers who complete the CDC reports. A California study found that 21 percent of women entering a drug treatment program reported having had sex with both men and women or with women exclusively. In this study, of women who had one or more female sexual partners since 1980, 76 percent were injection drug users (IDUs). A Kinsey Institute study of 400 lesbians found that 46 percent reported having sex with men, 88 percent reported having had vaginal sex with men, and 30 percent reported having had anal sex. Only 5 to 8 percent of individuals in these two groups reported regular use of condoms.

Recommendation

To avoid heterosexual bias in research, it is necessary to stress the confidentiality of participants and request information on sexual orientation. Language implying a heterosexual bias needs to be removed. Lesbian and gay researchers can help design studies, develop research questions, and make recommendations.

Issues for Future Research

- Research is needed to determine the rates of smoking, alcohol consumption, and other drug abuse behaviors among lesbians. The rates of HIV infection among lesbian IDUs compared with heterosexual women who are IDUs need to be investigated.

- Information is needed to determine if there are differences in treatment outcomes among lesbian, bisexual, and heterosexual women as well as treatment differences in terms of race and ethnicity. The characteristics of successful drug abuse programs in the lesbian community need to be identified.

- According to some research, lesbians are at higher risk of HIV infection than are heterosexual women. More research is needed on this risk factor and the epidemiology of HIV/AIDS among lesbians.

- Beliefs held by the lesbian community may indicate important areas of research. For example, one belief is that societal homophobia leads to increased drug abuse among lesbians; another is that alcohol use is high because, until recently, bars were the only social venue available to lesbians. A third belief is that the lack of treatment services sensitive to lesbians and gays has led to an increase in drug abuse.

HISPANIC WOMEN

Margarita Alegría, Ph.D.

Abstract

Dr. Alegría pointed out that there is a lack of research on Hispanic women who abuse drugs, but the information that does exist indicates that patterns of drug use and correlates of drug abuse vary among ethnic subgroups. She asserted that the current conceptual models were not adequate for understanding drug-related behaviors among Hispanic women. Multicausal models need to be investigated and should examine institutional, individual, and interpersonal factors, with an emphasis on institutional factors. Longitudinal studies are needed to understand the development of drug abuse in Hispanic women, its consequences, barriers for Hispanic women in obtaining drug treatment, treatment outcomes, and the effectiveness of treatment methods. More information is needed on the influence of acculturation level, social class, rural versus urban settings, and stressful life experiences on Hispanic women's abuse of drugs.

Current Knowledge

Many researchers agree that there is little understanding of the factors associated with drug abuse by Hispanic women. Most studies have included only a small proportion of Hispanics and omitted collecting data on sex differences. Recent national data on drug abuse have begun to reveal some sex differences and have provided descriptive information on drug abuse by Hispanic women.

- Hispanic women are as likely as white women to have used cocaine and as likely as blacks to have used crack or alcohol, but they are less likely than either group to have used cigarettes or marijuana.

- The use of drugs appears to vary among the three major Hispanic groups—Mexican-Americans, Puerto Ricans, and Cuban-Americans—and the correlates of drug abuse appear to vary significantly. It is not known whether the variations are because of cultural differences or other variables such as level of acculturation, social class, rural or urban setting, or stressful life experiences.

- There are methodological problems in studies that have been conducted on drug abuse by Hispanic women. For example, sex workers and incarcerated women have been excluded from studies. The underreporting of drug abuse is a potential problem because women fear losing their children. Self-administered questionnaires have presented problems for women of low literacy, and instruments have been used that were not designed or validated for use by Hispanic women. Cross-sectional study designs have been used that do not provide information about the development of drug abuse in Hispanic women.

- Current conceptual models are not adequate for understanding the drug abuse behaviors of Hispanic women because these models typically neglect unique variables such as family orientation, migration, loss of status within the community, and strong interpersonal networks. Models that focus on interpersonal, institutional, and community variables are needed so that social norms and constraints are examined and better understood; the institutional component is particularly important.

- Some correlates of drug abuse by Hispanic women have been identified, including hopelessness, depression, attitudes toward deviance, conduct problems, early sexual activity, low educational achievement, degree of religiosity, and boredom. Interpersonal factors identified as correlates include nontraditional family values, friends and relatives who use drugs, family discord, and social isolation. At the social and community levels, the correlates of drug abuse are acculturation, urban-rural differences, social class, and drug availability.

- Little attention has been given to the nature of and access to drug treatment for Hispanic women. Some studies report underuse of treatment services by Hispanics, whereas others find

Hispanics are overrepresented. Most treatment interventions and strategies used with Hispanic women have been based on models developed for Hispanic men. There is a dearth of knowledge about the effectiveness of drug treatment services delivered to Hispanic women.

- Researchers have found important differences among racial and ethnic minority groups regarding their denial of the need for drug treatment or their perception of benefits from treatment. Hispanic drug abusers who had been arrested were significantly less likely than whites to have received drug abuse treatment or to recognize that they needed such treatment.

Recent Findings

Dr. Alegría observed that little is known about what drug treatment programs are most appropriate for Hispanic women. She described the findings of research with inner-city Puerto Rican women who abused drugs, which was conducted to determine to what extent social service variables affected their willingness to seek treatment.

- The women reported that their most urgent needs were for jobs, housing, social services, help for their children, and drug rehabilitation. Health services usually responded only to women's physical health needs, without attention to coexisting problems such as depression, physical and sexual abuse, or domestic violence.

- There was a lack of coordination among Government service agencies that allowed women to fall through the cracks and miss intervention opportunities. In addition, eligibility requirements for entering drug treatment or rehabilitation programs excluded many women. Requirements such as a stable home environment, a medicaid card, or absence of a criminal record marginalize women and keep them out of institutional programs.

- Barriers to drug treatment were related more to the agencies that were to provide treatment than to women's personal factors. These barriers included rejection by providers, lack of available services or poor quality services, programs too short in duration to be effective, and lack of transitional programs.

Issues for Future Research

- A multicausal model of drug abuse in Hispanic women needs to be investigated and should include individual, interpersonal, institutional, and community factors. More research is needed on the influence of acculturation level, social class, rural and urban settings, and stressful life experience on drug abuse in ethnic subgroups of Hispanic women.

- The correlates to drug abuse among Hispanic women need to be examined; they include hopelessness, depression, attitudes toward deviance, conduct problems, early sexual activity, low educational achievement, degree of religiosity, and boredom. Other factors requiring attention include nontraditional family values, friends and family who use drugs, family discord, social isolation, and drug availability.

- Longitudinal studies of Hispanic women are needed to help explain the developmental course and consequences of drug abuse in this population.

- Research is needed on the problems, needs, and access barriers experienced by Hispanic women who seek drug treatment. What is their rate of participation, and what factors motivate Hispanic women to seek treatment? How effective is drug treatment for them? Another hypothesis to test is whether sustained drug problems and the lack of effective interventions cause an inordinate number of Hispanic women to be imprisoned.

- There seems to be a dearth of knowledge about the effectiveness of drug treatment services delivered to Hispanic women, and more emphasis is needed on understanding what services enhance clinical and functional outcomes. Studies should seek to identify successful treatments in community-based settings with parameters for what would be considered successful outcomes.

- The quality of programs needs to be assessed to identify the service elements that can improve clinical and functional outcomes for Hispanic women. Conceptual models cannot remain focused on the individual and personal variables associated with a woman's prolonged use of drugs.

RESEARCH NEEDS OF AMERICAN INDIAN WOMEN

Pamela Jumper-Thurman, Ph.D.

Abstract

Dr. Thurman presented research information about the health of American Indian women and alcohol and other drug abuse. The needs of American Indian women vary according to tribe and reservation, yet many women are affected greatly by alcoholism, other drug abuse, and poverty. The age-adjusted mortality rates for tuberculosis, alcoholism, and accidents among American Indians are more than twice that for all other races in the United States. There is little information on rates of crime and violence among American Indians, but some evidence suggests that alcohol abuse is highly associated with criminal and deviant behavior. Research is needed to identify drug abuse prevention, intervention, and treatment strategies that meet the needs of American Indian women, but researchers must work in partnership with American Indian tribes to ensure community participation and support.

Information From the Research Literature

American Indians are a diverse group, and women from various tribes and regions respond to problems differently. Drug abuse behavior varies according to tribal region, and each tribe has its own way of evaluating community needs. To be effective, drug abuse interventions must be consistent with the community's understanding of its needs.

- Many American Indian women are single parents, and they sometimes support the children of friends and relatives. Many American Indian women are affected greatly by alcoholism, other drug abuse, poverty, limited opportunities, and violence, and it has been reported that some American Indian children have learning disabilities and are undernourished, neglected, and unsupervised.

- Nineteen percent of American Indian families receive public assistance, compared with 5 percent of the total U.S. population. Thirty-one percent of American Indians earn salaries below the poverty level, compared with 13 percent of all other races in the United States. As many as 75 percent of reservation households are headed by women.

127

- The Indian Health Service reports that the age-adjusted mortality rates for some diseases and conditions are higher among American Indians than among all other races in the United States. For example, mortality from tuberculosis is 520 percent greater among American Indians, and the mortality rate from alcoholism is 433 percent greater. The mortality rate for American Indian women from accidents, including those involving motor vehicles, is twice the rate for women of all other races in the United States. Homicide and suicide rates also are higher among American Indians, and a significant number die at an early age.

- Anecdotal reports from physicians serving American Indian tribes have expressed concern about high rates of sexually transmitted diseases and increasing HIV infection rates.

- Although there is little information on rates of crime and violence in the American Indian population, existing data show that alcohol use is highly associated with criminal and deviant behavior.

- The use of cigarettes and inhalants among American Indian females is high, and cigarette use is higher among females than among males.

- Alcohol use appears to be a problem for many American Indian tribes and reservations. National comparative studies across racial and ethnic groups indicate that American Indian adolescents have the highest rates of alcohol use when compared with other adolescents. Alcohol use is slightly higher among adolescent males than females, and high rates of fetal alcohol syndrome are reported in some areas.

Issues for Future Research

- Research projects with American Indian populations must be developed in equal partnership. The research goals must be consistent with the community's understanding of its needs and must offer something of value to the community that will improve living conditions and empower tribes. American Indian women are reluctant to participate in programs that operate for 3 to 4 years and then disappear.

- Research is needed on the barriers to drug treatment faced by American Indian women and on strategies for prevention, intervention, and treatment that will meet their needs. Better health education and outreach strategies also are needed.

- Given the anecdotal information on violence, victimization, and alcoholism among American Indian women, a continuing database is needed to track mental health information, including data on posttraumatic stress disorder, and to track trends in drug abuse and crime in the American Indian population.

CROSSCUTTING ISSUES PANEL DISCUSSION

The discussion presented below followed presentations by members of the Crosscutting Issues Panel: Dr. Brissett-Chapman, Ms. Plumb, Dr. Alegría, and Dr. Jumper-Thurman.

Dr. Nan Vandenberg: It is assumed that 25 to 30 percent of lesbians are mothers, but we have not heard anything about drug abuse programs for these women. I challenge those in research to recognize the population of drug-abusing lesbian mothers in designing prevention and intervention programs. In the past 10 or 15 years there has been an increase in the number of lesbian or bisexual women who are having children through artificial insemination. I want to underscore the continuum of sexual behavior in the sense that someone who may have been heterosexual at one point in time may later have sex with other women, and then return to having sex with men. Second, we need to realize that the workplace might be an important place to direct drug abuse prevention programs at gays and lesbians because many "come out" only in their 20s or 30s. Government-sponsored research on drug abuse needs to collect and analyze data on sexual orientation.

Unidentified Audience Member: I am in the Office of AIDS Research, and my Internet communications around the world indicate that few lesbians are concerned about HIV; they point to the lack of research [that would substantiate the danger]. I have been in a number of studies as a control because I am a healthy female. No one ever asks about my sexual orientation, but when they wonder why I am not on birth control, I explain that I am a lesbian.

Ms. Plumb: I want to underscore the point that the white lesbian and gay community has little contact with lesbians and gays from communities of color, so those communities have had difficulty dealing with white lesbians and gays. Few studies include lesbian and bisexual women of color; therefore, the intersection of race and sexual orientation probably has not been evaluated.

Dr. Brissett-Chapman: I want to comment from the African-American perspective. I believe the African-American community has been researched intrusively for information that does not always lead to particular program or policy responses. The more questions we ask of women, for example, at the shelter, the more responsible we must be in understanding what effect this information may have on women in the community. How will we address the issues of stigma often associated with lesbian women of color, and how will we support these women in the community?

Dr. Coryl Jones: Marj Plumb has offered to help researchers gain access to this population of women in terms of drug abuse research. There are cultural, ethnic, and language problems in our studies that affect communication between investigators and research subjects. We must translate our research instruments to ensure they mean the same thing in the languages of everyone involved and to make sure that desired information is communicated between investigators and research subjects. We must add communications skills to our research agenda.

Closing Session

CONCLUDING REMARKS

David J. Mactas
Director
Center for Substance Abuse Treatment

Mr. Mactas reported that he is committed to having the Center for Substance Abuse Treatment (CSAT) collaborate with NIDA, the National Institute on Alcohol Abuse and Alcoholism, and other research organizations. He described the following future initiatives of CSAT:

- CSAT will work with the National Institute of Child Health and Human Development, which has developed a manual on treatment approaches for women who abuse alcohol and other drugs. CSAT also will collaborate on preparing a comprehensive model of care for treatment of women and their children.

- As mandated by Congress, CSAT will support drug abuse treatment research and services for women and children. CSAT funds 65 residential and 12 outpatient drug abuse treatment programs that serve mothers with children younger than 10.

- CSAT will respond to its constituency and help people who face barriers to treatment and who rely on Government support to obtain treatment. Efforts may include scholarships, advocacy, and the acquisition of new resources.

Mr. Mactas invited the audience to speak with him and his staff about CSAT's programs in more detail after the session.

TOWARD THE DEVELOPMENT OF A DRUG ABUSE RESEARCH AGENDA ON THE HEALTH OF WOMEN

Richard A. Millstein
Deputy Director
National Institute on Drug Abuse

Mr. Millstein thanked conference participants for sharing their knowledge about women and drug abuse and in this way helping shape NIDA's research agenda. He observed that conference speakers had identified the wide information gap on women and drug abuse and identified new research ideas to bridge that gap. The results of research on men cannot be confidently and safely generalized to women.

Mr. Millstein reviewed NIDA's efforts to study drug abuse among women and sex differences. Although many previous studies have focused on pregnant women and their offspring, the focus is expanding to include women of all ages. He described the following NIDA initiatives on women:

- In June 1993 NIDA undertook a technical review on drug abuse and HIV infection and their effect on women and children.

- NIDA issued two program announcements in 1993 seeking applications for research on the etiology, consequences, and behavioral pharmacology of female drug abuse and treatment for women of childbearing age and children. Some NIDA program announcements on HIV focused indirectly on women's issues, such as partner notification of HIV-infected drug abusers and strategies to reduce high-risk sexual practices among drug abusers.

- In June 1994 NIDA held a technical review on methodological issues related to the etiology and consequences of drug abuse among women.

- NIDA has produced brochures, videotapes, and NIDA Capsules with information on women and drug abuse.

NIDA has provided many grants to fund research programs that focus on women's issues and sex differences, but Mr. Millstein noted that more research is needed. Research on women and drug abuse is one of NIDA's key priority areas. The Institute wants to determine the biological and behavioral sex differences that need to be addressed and the effectiveness of various drug abuse prevention and treatment programs. Mr. Millstein urged conference participants to apply for NIDA grants, and he asked clinicians and practitioners to make recommendations regarding NIDA's research agenda.

Mr. Millstein summarized the questions and issues identified during the conference that are important to developing NIDA's research agenda on drug abuse and women's health. The following are illustrative of those he addressed:

Prevention and Treatment

- Because the rates of anxiety and affective disorders, which are possible precursors to drug abuse and dependence, are higher among women than among men, research is needed on better treatment of these disorders in women. Research also is needed on the consequences of providing or withholding such treatment, particularly for pregnant women.

- Prevention and treatment programs should be designed to address specific research-based risk factors among women, including childhood physical and sexual abuse, victimization, posttraumatic stress disorder, and partner violence.

- The sex differences found in drug abuse treatment research include legal barriers and women's fears about losing their children; lack of comprehensive health care services; lack of access to child care services, perinatal programs, and prenatal care; inadequate vocational education; dangerous physical environments and housing; low self-esteem; and feelings of hopelessness and depression that require mental health counseling and treatment.

- Research is needed on how to improve the recruitment and retention of women in research studies. Women have been found to be less likely than men to accept random study assignments. Women may respond to treatment strategies that are different from those that men respond to and may respond less to treatments that are successful with men. Strategies that may be more successful with women than men include comprehensive services and treatments that address violence, victimization, stress, and health and social services case management.

- Diverse care models and integrated approaches are needed to link health care, drug treatment, and HIV services. Research on health care services should be broad and incorporate not just drug abuse treatment but also AIDS treatment, primary care and access to care, and use of services.

- Information is needed on the effectiveness of drug abuse-related program approaches for different racial and ethnic subgroups and other subgroups of women. Specific factors such as sex-related issues, violence, racism, sexual orientation, and program philosophies also need to be examined for their effect on drug abuse prevention and treatment approaches. Examination is needed of the combined effects of social, cultural, economic, environmental, and genetic factors.

- The definition of substance abuse with regard to licit and illicit drugs should be reexamined, discussed, and clarified. Discussion also is needed to reach agreement on the definition of successful drug treatment outcomes.

- Discussion is needed on the appropriate use of the term "relapse" in relation to drug abuse treatment. Would it be more appropriate to use the term "recurrence," an expected or normal return of symptoms, than "relapse," the return of a disease? Recurrence is the term used by clinicians when referring to other chronic disorders such as hypertension or diabetes.

- The drug abuse research and treatment communities need to work with Congress, the executive branch, the medical community (including obstetricians, gynecologists, and pediatricians), the academic community, and the media to educate the public about the importance of drug abuse prevention, intervention, and treatment.

- The complex issues related to women's enrollment in clinical trials to determine drug efficacy, including the enrollment of pregnant women, should be discussed and resolved.

Epidemiology

- The role of sex differences in vulnerability to drug abuse requires study, as does the progression from drug use to abuse and dependence. What are the implications of these sex differences for prevention and treatment strategies? This work holds enormous promise and will further understanding about dopamine system regulation and drug use.

- Replication is needed of the initial findings of research on the intergenerational transmission of smoking from women who smoke during pregnancy to their female offspring. At the same time, researchers must avoid judging or blaming women for their behaviors and fetal outcomes.

- Information is needed on the different risk factors for HIV infection among women and men. Drug abuse is a vector for AIDS in women more often than it is in men. What is the reason for this difference?

- More research is needed on the epidemiology of drug abuse and AIDS among various populations of women. For example, there is little epidemiologic information on drug abuse among lesbians, and therefore there is little information about the epidemiology of AIDS and drug abuse prevention and treatment for this population.

Etiology

- Research is needed on the etiology of drug abuse and the child and adolescent precursors and personality pathways that lead to drug use and progression to abuse and dependence. Research is needed on protective factors, resiliency, invulnerability, and prevention of drug abuse.

- Important research and prevention issues should be addressed relating to intergenerational models of violence and of alcohol and other drug problems. Family dynamics and their effect on drug abuse also need attention.

- More information is needed on the efficacy of strategies to reduce the harmful consequences of drug use. Attempts must be made to reach a consensus on the role of reductions in drug use and other negative outcomes and consequences (short of drug abstinence) as successful treatment outcomes.

Biological and Behavioral Mechanisms

- Research is needed on the biological and behavioral mechanisms of drug abuse, including cocaine's effect on reproductive functioning, the effect of the menstrual cycle on cocaine self-administration, sex differences in male and female responses to serotoninergic transmission, and sex-specific considerations in the use of psychoactive medications.

- The implications of recent findings on biological and behavioral approaches to drug abuse intervention must be examined.

Consequences

- There are sex differences in the median survival time from AIDS diagnosis to death. Do women present with the disease later than men, and if so, why? Why are women underscreened for HIV infection and drug abuse compared with men?

- Research suggests that AZT is more likely to be offered to men than women. What are the implications for women, and what are the barriers to treatment?

- Among women taking AZT, 8.3 percent gave birth to neonates with HIV infection versus 25.5 percent among women not taking AZT. Has this information been incorporated into drug treatment and demonstration programs? What changes in medical practice have occurred?

- It is important to examine further the association of alcohol and other drug use with mental health problems, poor pregnancy outcomes, and high-risk sexual behaviors. What are the social and behavioral consequences to women who have low self-esteem? How can social supports and protective factors be strengthened?

Crosscutting Research Issues

- Women are a heterogeneous group, and different subgroups will require different strategies for drug abuse prevention, treatment, and research. Information on women of different racial and ethnic minority groups, ages, and sexual orientations must be collected and analyzed to determine what differences in strategy will be needed for drug abuse prevention and treatment in different subgroups.

- There has been a proliferation of agencies with drug abuse programs, including NIDA; Substance Abuse and Mental Health Services Administration (SAMHSA); Center for Substance Abuse Treatment; Center for Substance Abuse Prevention; National Cancer Institute; National Heart, Lung, and Blood Institute; Centers for Disease Control and Prevention; National Institute of Child Health and Human Development; National Institute of Mental Health; National Institute on Alcohol Abuse and Alcoholism; and Indian Health Service, among others. Multiple partnerships among Government programs and agencies are needed so that the responsibility for conducting research and addressing issues is shared. Coordination is needed to ensure that agencies will be held accountable for implementing comprehensive initiatives that address the needs of the whole person.

- Several conference speakers recommended more training for both researchers and providers. NIDA has a role in research training, and SAMHSA and the Health Resources and Services Administration are the agencies most likely to be involved in clinician training.

- The dissemination and application of research findings is key; therefore, models are needed of the most effective methods of disseminating information and encouraging the application of research information in clinical practice.

- More women researchers are needed to ensure that questions related to sex differences are not overlooked. Researchers from diverse population groups must be supported, including women of color and women of different sexual orientations.

Mr. Millstein concluded his remarks by thanking the conference organizers, presenters, and participants, and he again encouraged participants to contact NIDA with their input into the direction and priorities of this research agenda.

Conference Speakers

Margarita Alegría, Ph.D.
Associate Professor
Center for Sociomedical Research
  and Evaluation
Graduate School of Public Health
Medical Sciences Campus
University of Puerto Rico
P.O. Box 365067
San Juan, PR 00936-5067

D. Caroline Blanchard, Ph.D.
Professor
Department of Anatomy
Bekesy Laboratory of
  Neurobiology
John A. Burns School of Medicine
University of Hawaii, Manoa
1993 East-West Road
Honolulu, HI 96822-2359

Susan J. Blumenthal, M.D.,
  M.P.A.
Deputy Assistant Secretary for
  Health (Women's Health)
U.S. Department of Health and
  Human Services
Office on Women's Health
Humphrey Building, Room 730-B
200 Independence Avenue, S.W.
Washington, DC 20201

Sheryl Brissett-Chapman, Ed.D.,
  A.C.S.W., L.I.C.S.W.
Executive Director
Baptist Home for Children and
  Families
6301 Greentree Road
Bethesda, MD 20817

Judith S. Brook, Ed.D.
Professor of Community Medicine
Mount Sinai School of Medicine
Box 1044A
One Gustave L. Levy Place
New York, NY 10029

Shirley D. Coletti, D.H.L.
President
Operation PAR, Inc.
Pinellas Business Center,
  Administrative Offices
Suite 1000
10901-C Roosevelt Boulevard
St. Petersburg, FL 33716

R. Lorraine Collins, Ph.D.
Senior Research Scientist
Research Institute on Addictions
1021 Main Street
Buffalo, NY 14203

Linda B. Cottler, Ph.D.
Associate Professor of
  Epidemiology in Psychiatry
Department of Psychiatry
Washington University School
  of Medicine
40 North Kingshighway
  Boulevard, Suite 4
St. Louis, MO 63108

Loretta P. Finnegan, M.D.
Director
Women's Health Initiative
Office of the Director
National Institutes of Health
Room 6C12
7550 Wisconsin Avenue
Bethesda, MD 20892-9112

Neil E. Grunberg, Ph.D.
Professor
Department of Medical and
  Clinical Psychology
Uniformed Services University
  of the Health Sciences
4301 Jones Bridge Road
Bethesda, MD 20814-4799

Pamela Jumper-Thurman, Ph.D.
Research Associate
Tri-Ethnic Center for Prevention
  Research
Department of Psychology
Colorado State University
Clark C138A
Fort Collins, CO 80523

Stephen R. Kandall, M.D.
Professor of Pediatrics
Albert Einstein College of
  Medicine
Chief
Division of Neonatology
Beth Israel Medical Center
7 Baird Hall
First Avenue and 16th Street
New York, NY 10003

Denise B. Kandel, Ph.D.
Professor of Public Health in
  Psychiatry
College of Physicians and
  Surgeons
Columbia University
Chief
Division of Epidemiology of
  Substance Abuse
New York State Psychiatric
  Institute
722 West 168th Street, Box 20
New York, NY 10032

Dean G. Kilpatrick, Ph.D.
Professor
National Crime Victims Research
  and Treatment Center
Department of Psychiatry and
  Behavioral Sciences
Medical University of South
  Carolina
171 Ashley Avenue
Charleston, SC 29425-0742

Mary Jeanne Kreek, M.D.
Professor
Head
Laboratory on the Biology of
  Addictive Diseases
Rockefeller University
1230 York Avenue
New York, NY 10021

Karol L. Kumpfer, Ph.D.
Associate Professor
Department of Health Education
Health Sciences Center
HPER N-215
University of Utah
Salt Lake City, UT 84112

Alan I. Leshner, Ph.D.
Director
National Institute on Drug Abuse
Parklawn Building, Room 10-05
5600 Fishers Lane
Rockville, MD 20857

David J. Mactas
Director
Center for Substance Abuse
  Treatment
Substance Abuse and Mental
  Health Services Administration
Rockwall II, Suite 615
5600 Fishers Lane
Rockville, MD 20857

Nancy K. Mello, Ph.D.
Professor of Psychology
  (Neuroscience)
Co-Director
Harvard Medical School
Alcohol and Drug Abuse
  Research Center
McLean Hospital
115 Mill Street
Belmont, MA 02178

Kathleen R. Merikangas, Ph.D.
Professor of Epidemiology and
  Psychiatry
Departments of Psychiatry and
  Epidemiology
Genetic Epidemiology Research
  Unit
Yale University School of
  Medicine
40 Temple Street, Suite 7B
New Haven, CT 06510-3223

Brenda A. Miller, Ph.D.
Acting Director
Research Institute on Addictions
1021 Main Street
Buffalo, NY 14203-1016

Richard A. Millstein
Deputy Director
National Institute on Drug Abuse
5600 Fishers Lane, Room 10-05
Rockville, MD 20857

Karla Moras, Ph.D.
Assistant Professor of Psychology
  and Psychiatry
Center for Psychotherapy
  Research
University of Pennsylvania
Seventh Floor
3600 Market Street
Philadelphia, PA 19104-2640

Adeline Nyamathi, R.N., Ph.D.,
  F.A.A.N.
Associate Professor
School of Nursing
University of California,
  Los Angeles
10833 LeConte Avenue
Los Angeles, CA 90024-6918

Lynn M. Paltrow, J.D.
Reproductive Policy Attorney
45 West 10th Street
New York, NY 10011

Vivian W. Pinn, M.D.
Associate Director for Research
  on Women's Health
Director
Office of Research on Women's
  Health
National Institutes of Health
Building 1, Room 201
9000 Rockville Pike
Bethesda, MD 20892

Marjorie J. Plumb, M.N.A.
Director of Public Policy
Gay and Lesbian Medical
  Association
459 Fulton Street, Suite 107
San Francisco, CA 94102

David C.S. Roberts, Ph.D.
Professor
Department of Psychology
Life Sciences Research Centre
Carleton University
1125 Colonel By Drive
Ottawa, Ontario K1S 5B6
CANADA

Rafaela R. Robles, Ed.D.
Senior Scientist
Research Institute
Mental Health and Anti-
  Addiction Services
  Administration
Center for Sociomedical Research
Medical Sciences Campus
University of Puerto Rico
Center for Addiction Studies
School of Medicine
Universidad Central de Caribe
P.O. Box 21414
San Juan, PR 00928-1414

Marsha Rosenbaum, Ph.D.
Director
The Lindesmith Center-West
2233 Lombard Street
San Francisco, CA 94123

Kathy Sanders-Phillips, Ph.D.
Associate Professor
Department of Pediatrics
School of Medicine
University of California,
   Los Angeles
5120 Goldleaf Circle, Suite 380
Los Angeles, CA 90056

Sidney Schnoll, M.D., Ph.D.
Professor
Departments of Internal Medicine
   and Psychiatry
Chairman
Division of Substance Abuse
   Medicine
Medical College of Virginia
   Hospitals
Box 980109
Richmond, VA 23298-0109

Peter A. Selwyn, M.D., M.P.H.
Associate Director
AIDS Program
Associate Professor of Medicine,
   Epidemiology, and Public Health
Yale University School of Medicine
135 College Street, Suite 323
New Haven, CT 06510

Jacqueline Wallen, Ph.D., M.S.W.
Associate Professor
Department of Family Studies
University of Maryland
1204 Marie Mount Hall
College Park, MD 20742

James R. Woods, Jr., M.D.
Professor
Obstetrics and Gynecology
Director
Maternal-Fetal Medicine
Strong Memorial Hospital
601 Elmwood Avenue, Box 668
Rochester, NY 14642-8668